I'M ALIVE

Courage, Hope, and a Miracle

Duke Pieper

with Jim Bruton

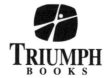

TRIUMPH
BOOKS

Library of Congress Cataloging-in-Publication Data

Pieper, Duke, 1993–

I'm alive : courage, hope, and a miracle / Duke Pieper with Jim Bruton ;
 foreword by Lou Nanne.
   pages cm
 ISBN 978-1-62937-135-1 (paperback)
 1. Pieper, Duke, 1993—Health. 2. Brain—Surgery. 3. Hockey
   players—Minnesota—Biography.   I. Bruton, James H., 1945– II. Title.
 RD594.P54 2015
 617.4'81—dc23

                                                    2015020065

This book is available in quantity at special discounts for your group or organization. For further information, contact:

Triumph Books LLC
   814 North Franklin Street
   Chicago, Illinois 60610
   (312) 337-0747
   www.triumphbooks.com

Printed in U.S.A.

ISBN: 978-1-62937-135-1

Design by Amy Carter

Photos courtesy of the author unless otherwise indicated

I have wanted to write this book, my story of what happened to me, for a long time. I write it in the hopes that it may provide comfort and guidance to those who have faced a life-changing experience, or perhaps just to inspire or motivate people in some other way. It is one of the most important things I have ever done and means the world to me.

I dedicate this book to the three most important people in my life: my wonderful mom, my exceptional dad, and my incredible sister. I love you from the depths of my heart.

CONTENTS

FOREWORD

Sometimes we cross paths with an individual who leaves an indelible impression on us because of his or her unique personality and story. Duke Pieper is one of those people.

As a youngster, Duke demonstrated great hockey potential. I first saw him play in Edina, and he was an excellent talent. In seventh and eighth grades he played at Shattuck–St. Mary's, a noted private school that has produced many top NHL players. This is where I first watched him in action. As a freshman, he made the varsity at Hill-Murray, a perennial high school hockey power in the state of Minnesota.

Just before his first game, he suffered a brain bleed. Given only a 5 percent chance of living through surgery, he miraculously survived. His entire life changed in an instant, but a new life began for him.

This book explores his drive, his ability to inspire others, his commitment, his confidence, and most of all, his attitude. This is what led him to succeed where many other people would have quit. He has the characteristics that any one of us would love to have, and a mind-set to succeed in the face of overpowering adversity that is seldom seen. Anyone would be proud and feel privileged to have a son, brother, uncle, husband, or friend like him.

You will be captivated by the manner in which he overcame his challenges and marvel at his growth as a leader among his peers.

—Lou Nanne,
Olympian, Minnesota Gophers
All-American, and Minnesota
North Stars player, coach, general
manager, and president

COAUTHOR'S NOTE

I have to be honest. I don't know how you respectfully, thoughtfully, and accurately convey the magnificent story of this courageously gifted young man, Duke Pieper. There are too many parts full of passion and emotion, too many tears, too many shattered goals. His passion to inspire and his relentless spirit are infectious.

How do you give ample attention and adequate recognition for his accomplishments in bringing his life back to some form of normalcy? The only way is to have Duke tell his story in his own words, and to leave in all the painful, heartbreaking, and joyous details.

This is the true story of what happened to Duke Pieper, and how he has been able to utilize his crushing, life-changing experience to motivate him in the depths of his heart and soul—something unimaginable to anyone who has not faced this type of peril.

His account takes us with him on the ice at Hill-Murray School— his triumph of making the varsity hockey team of the reigning state champs as a ninth-grader, and the loneliest moment of his life as he takes his skates off in the back of the locker room for the last time. We are with him through his arduous fight for survival from a destructive brain lesion as he battles to breathe, walk, talk, and live again.

How do you recover from having your life's dreams gone forever? How do you motivate yourself to enjoy life again? How do you find meaning in misfortune?

Duke Pieper will never play hockey again. What looked to be a promising and long career in the sport was all over for him at the age of 15. And yet for Duke it was a new beginning. He understands. He gets it. He has figured out at such an early age what the important things in life are. And yet, his journey has just begun.

Duke holds nothing back in telling his story. We descend with him to the depths of his darkest moments, and celebrate his accomplishments alongside him. It is an amazing story indeed—one filled with sadness and utter joy. In his short life span, he has already endured more than most people will in a lifetime.

While moving through the most difficult stages of his life, he has developed lifelong friendships. Murray Eaves, Bill Lechner, Paul Otto, Pat Schafhauser, Chris Bergeron, Cal Dietz, and Larry Hendrickson graciously agreed to be part of this book because of their admiration for Duke and his passion to succeed against all obstacles. Duke greatly values the role that each of them has played helping him to face unimaginable obstacles. Through these men's words, it is evident that Duke has given back to them in kind.

Duke Pieper is an incredible human being, a young man who faced overwhelming devastation. Rather than be discouraged by unimaginable circumstances, he has found meaning and purpose in it. He is no less than an inspiration to us all.

—Jim Bruton

What Is Happening to Me?

This happened to me. At least I think it did. Sometimes it seems too crazy to be real. I didn't know it at the time, but it was the beginning of the end of life as I knew it.

There is a time in my life—approximately two months, give or take a few days—that I only vaguely remember. It was after my first surgery, while I was hospitalized. I had a lot of dreams (both asleep and awake) and a great deal of confusion. There was make-believe stuff, at least I think it was make-believe, that came in and out of my mind. From what I have been told by my mom and dad, I did some pretty bizarre things. I would call out to hockey players as if we were on the ice in the middle of a game. I would *yell* at them—my own teammates. *"Pass the puck! Shoot! Shoot!"* Sometimes I would yell as if we were in a football game—*"You have position. Run! Run!"*—giving instructions.

• • •

11

My mom told me that sometimes I would jump over my bed as if I was going over hockey boards to get on the ice. Why did I do this? I didn't have an answer. These things just *happened*.

. . .

I had dreams that didn't make any sense at all. Very early on during this time I recall being in the intensive care unit at the hospital. I remember it like it was yesterday. I was sitting on my bed, and I felt like I was elevated. I felt top-heavy. I thought I was going to fall head over heels. It was a strange feeling. I recall hearing a voice saying, "I'm your mom. I'm your mom." I kept asking her over and over again who she was. I didn't believe that she was who she said she was. *I didn't know her.*

In some ways I understood that this woman in my room was my mom, but I was confused. Actually, at times I thought that she was a bumblebee. I know that doesn't make any sense, but that was the reality for me at the time. I couldn't put two and two together. I actually was convinced that my mom was a bumblebee. I was in trouble and I didn't know why.

There were other things that happened during this time, memories that might have been a dream or maybe really did occur. I think that some of them are true and that some are make-believe. Dreams, I guess, is the best word to describe them. Hallucinations? Maybe. I didn't know one from the other. I just couldn't tell the difference.

. . .

My bed was another problem for me. When I was in it, I felt as if everything below it was a pit. I was cold, too—very, very cold in my room. Other times I heard the roar of a helicopter engine over my head. It was there and the sounds were real. I never actually saw the helicopter, but I truly believed it was there. *"I can hear it. I can hear the helicopter. It's there, I know it is."* I never once saw it, though.

Looking back, I can't say exactly when all this happened or even what the right sequence is, but it was a very real part of what was going on with me at the time. It was and is confusing, but the clarity of those memories is undeniable; it all felt so real.

• • •

I can recall at one point being in a wheelchair after one of my surgeries. I was sitting in front of one of those inflatable plastic thingamajigs that you see in people's yards during the holidays. It may have been some kind of a blow-up snow globe. But inside of it was a person. I know what you're thinking—*This can't be real*—but it seemed that way to me. It was in the late fall, near Christmas, and the figure was some kind of character with a Christmas connection. I have trouble describing it, but it was very real to me.

I just stared at it for the longest time. My dad had put me in front of it and I was mad at him for putting me there. I didn't want to look at this thing, whatever it was. It disturbed me. Now, in my mind it was real, but maybe it *was* a dream. I just don't know. I won't ever know. There were so many things going on in my mind at the time that I couldn't decipher what was real and what wasn't.

• • •

Once I had to use the bathroom and a lady came in to assist me. She looked very strange to me—I thought she had a significant resemblance to a vampire. I'm not trying to be mean, but to me she really did look like a vampire. So when this person came into my room I asked her, "Who are you? Are you a vampire?" I know I said it out loud. In my "real" life that would not be me. I was taught to respect people and be kind and thoughtful. But back then, the fact was, I was neither. I said whatever came into my mind, period.

• • •

One day I found myself in a palace, a dirt palace, not one like you might see or imagine in the movies or in a fairy tale. I instinctively knew that it was a palace but it certainly wasn't nice. It had iron bars for doors. Down one corridor was a plate of food, and down another was basically nothing. I was eating the food and going through the rooms. And I wasn't there for a short time; I wandered through for a long time. These bizarre dreams seemed to last forever. What was happening to me? I was living in a world like nothing I had ever experienced before, and I didn't know how to come back.

• • •

I know now that I never really left the room, but even in the room I had a tough time. I saw millions of lightning bolts. They fell from the sky and each one jolted me. I *felt* them. But I could not find a way to make them stop.

These images went on for months, and each experience or hallucination or whatever you want to call it seemed to go on for days at a time. None of it made sense to me, but I understand now that it was all part of what I was going through. Something wrong in my head, with my brain, my mind.

• • •

All these dreams, hallucinations, or whatever you want to call them followed one of the worst moments in my life. It should have been one of the best, but instead it took a turn for the very worst. "Coach, this isn't going to happen for me tonight. I don't think I should play in the game." Those were my words to my coach before my first high school hockey game. I had made varsity as a freshman and it was our first game of the season. It was a huge accomplishment and I was so excited to take that stage for the first time. My friends, my family...everyone there in the stands to see it. I didn't know what was happening, but something just didn't feel right. I felt *off*. I couldn't have known that in that moment my hockey dream was over, or that I would enter a confusing and devastating journey into a mysterious world that I will never come to fully understand—a world of pain, make-believe, and lifelong ramifications.

CHAPTER 1

Just Your Average Family

I loved life as a young kid. I was always busy. I was like most kids, I suppose. I had fun and I made snow forts and I liked the winter months like every other boy in Minnesota. I also loved putting things together. I especially liked to play with LEGOs. I could put them together in a million different combinations. I had thousands of them. Every Christmas I would ask for more.

My parents, my sister, and I are a close-knit family. My dad is special. I get along with him really well. He is a big teddy bear, a big guy who can really squeeze you tight. He is a hard worker and a genuine person. He has always been there for me. Sure, I have to pick up after him once in a while, but nobody's perfect. We have a great relationship. Through all our hockey trips we spent a lot of time together. He has been a real mentor for me all my life.

He has an entrepreneurial spirit and likes to take on things and make them work. He likes to start new projects and has been pretty successful with all sorts of them over the years. Concerning this book project, I know he really wanted me to do it. He has been really encouraging. I think he feels that after everything that happened to me, I have a great story to tell. He feels like I had experiences that no one else had ever had before. He wants, like I do, for me to be able to share my story and provide help to others who have experienced tragedy in their lives.

My mom has always been there for me, too. We don't always have the same viewpoint on things and we get after each other from time to time, but that's okay. My mom is the details person. She is the one in our family who keeps track of things and gets things done. On the medical side, it has been my mom who is on top of things. She knows what is supposed to happen—especially with my medical problems. After my diagnosis she did all the research, and has been in charge of my physical therapy, my medications, and everything else. I depend on her, and she has never let me down. She never gave up, and was the driving force behind getting me through all this.

Mom was big in figure skating as a young woman and won some national awards. She coached figure skating, too, though she dropped most everything when I needed her. I would say that my mom has a huge heart; that became so obvious to me as she assisted me with every aspect of my new life, from coordinating with doctors and managing medications to keeping friends and family updated on my condition and generally handling all the day-to-day minutiae. She loves me deeply and has always been there for me. She watches out for me and is the one in our family who keeps it all together. Although my relationships with my parents are very different, it works for us. I feel very fortunate to have them both.

My sister, Jackie, and I get along great—when we're not playing jokes on one another. We trust each other implicitly, which is not something every guy can say about his sister. I think she is awesome. She often has been my confidant. Since she knows fashion and obviously knows about the female mind, I have checked in with her for some sisterly advice from time to time. She is also a great hockey player in her own right; she even played hockey in high school for me! She is currently on a hockey scholarship out at Merrimack College in Massachusetts. I have always joked with her that everything she has ever learned about hockey came from me. As you would expect, she has a little difference of opinion on that matter.

Jackie really took my medical problems to heart. I know it was extremely hard on her—not least of all because all of our parents' attention was focused on me during my recovery. She is a strong person and I admire her for that. We have a close relationship, and she has been there for me every step of the way. I hope she knows I will always be there for her, too.

We make a pretty great family, if you ask me. Though I can't forget the other members who make up our household. One of the real loves of my life as a young kid—and even today—has been my dogs. I am honestly convinced that having a dog gives a person a very different perspective on life. I guess it is the companionship, the love, and the loyalty that makes the relationship so special.

I was about eight when we got Pepsi, a Wheaten Terrier. My dad has always taken credit for the name, and usually I let him have it, but I know that I was the one who thought of Pepsi. My cousin had a dog named Cola, as in Coca-Cola. Well, once I heard that name, I knew that *our* dog had to be named Pepsi. It was just that simple.

Pepsi was a great dog, and absolutely spoiled rotten. Our connection was special. In fact, when I was in the hospital, my parents would bring Pepsi to the hospital to see me, and he knew exactly what room I was in. He would automatically go right to my room. He just knew. I always thought that was pretty neat. I was devastated when Pepsi passed away, but I will never forget him. He helped me through some very tough times.

Today we have two dogs. We have another Wheaten Terrier named Sprite—there we go with the pop names again—and we have Crosby, who is a miniature goldendoodle. My sister named Crosby after the great hockey player from the Pittsburgh Penguins, Sidney Crosby. They are both great pets who bring us pure joy.

As a family we have a lake place on Lake Alexandria near Brainerd, Minnesota. We have had it as long as I can remember. It has been in our family for generations. I love it up there. I always have something to do. Being the outdoor person that I am, I even enjoy cutting the grass and doing other yard work. I'm not much of a fisherman or hunter, so that doesn't occupy any of my time, but I really enjoy tubing, Jet Skiing, wakeboarding, and riding my motorcycle. These things come a little less easily for me now, admittedly.

My mom was a figure skater and she had me on ice skates when I was very young. I was terrible. I had no balance, so I didn't like it much. Hockey was kind of a pain in the butt for me. It was the equipment. I hated it. I hated putting on my skates, the pads; the discomfort of it all was too much and I complained a lot. I mean *a lot*. In fact, my parents actually had me sit out a year! It was a good call on their part, because I came around. Soon putting on a pair of skates became like putting on a pair of shoes to me. It all fit, and it fit better each time I got on the ice. Before long, hockey was a huge part of my life. I loved the game. I loved the sport. I loved the action, the competition, being with my teammates and coaches; it was my life! It was all I thought about each and every day. I was totally consumed by it.

There is something about the way it makes me feel. I feel a warmth inside when I think about the game, when I sit down to put my skates on, when I think about getting ready to play. Every single aspect of the game is a major thrill for me. Even the breeze you get in your face when you skate down the ice fascinates me. I enjoy the smell from the ice arena, seeing the fans in the stands, knowing my parents are at the game. I can't get enough of it.

The game gives me this incredible awesome feeling all over my body. I get chills down my back thinking about an upcoming game, thinking about the competition and winning. It is, in reality, tough to actually explain how it feels. There is just a connection that I have with the sport. It's tough to put it into words that do it justice; it is a connection unlike any other.

I have often thought about the difference in the sports that I am accustomed to playing and have come to the conclusion that there really is nothing else like hockey. Other sports have dead spots, time between plays, time between pitches, slowdown of play, those kinds of game aspects. Not hockey. It is constantly in motion, always something going on. The speed of the game is unbelievable. The action is superb. There is always something happening.

As I look back to the past, I know with my injury and all that has happened to me, I truly believe that parts of the game, even off the ice, have kept me going, kept my spirits up. The game has taught me to be in terrific condition, taught me to work out and stay sharp. Now that I cannot play anymore, still those parts of the game have stayed with me. Even with my disabilities I try to stay in top physical condition. Hockey has taught me that.

The game brought to me a belief that you have to always go out on the ice and do your very best or the game will pass you by. This has stayed with me. Without that drive that I learned, and the competitiveness, I would not be where I am today. I might have given up on all my problems and settled into a life of paralysis, a life of letting my physical handicaps take me down. I would be without the drive, the fight, and the "never give up" attitude.

I have also learned things like the importance of being on time. And I don't mean being five minutes early, because that is late. I mean getting there a half hour ahead, maybe an hour ahead of when you are supposed to be there, to get ready, get your mind right, and prepare yourself for the greatest game in the world.

There is a difference in playing inside and outside. Forget the actual game for a minute and think about playing outdoors on a pond or manufactured rink. Playing with my buddies in those settings is the best. The ice is kind of rugged, nobody keeps score, I cannot put words on the paper to describe it. There is nothing like it. You enjoy the weather, the chill in the air, the friendship; all to enjoy and become engulfed by.

And then the indoor arenas, the games, the fans, the competitiveness, the lights, the boards, the ice, the public address announcer, the scoreboards; *awesome* is the only word to characterize it. It gets my juices flowing just describing it and thinking about it.

My love was to play defense. I was a pretty tough player and I had a few fights in games, even though it is not allowed. I was really an aggressive player and found so much of the game that excited me. When I would score a goal, it was mind-boggling. When our goalie would make a big save, it was thrilling. A great fake or a perfect pass made the game worthwhile and kept the adrenaline flow at its peak. I could go on forever about every aspect of the game. It is emblazoned in me, a part of me.

I never wanted a game to end. I wanted to keep playing, shooting, passing, checking, and could hardly wait for the next time. I never had to concentrate on the ice. I never had to give any thought to what I was supposed to do with the puck, whom I was supposed to pass to; it all just came so natural to me. I never had to think about what I was supposed to do next. Never happened. The game fit me like the equipment. I loved it.

It seemed as if I was always doing something related to hockey. First there was the Mini-Mites, then the Mites, the Squirts, the Peewees, the Bantams, and then high school hockey. I played at all levels and was told that I was an exceptionally good player.

Initially when I started playing organized hockey, I wanted to be a goalie. The only problem was, I was terrible at it. More pucks seemed to go in than what I stopped. My dad once asked me, "Duke, why are you letting all these pucks get by you? Why are you letting in so many goals?" And I remember I told him, "Dad, I want my teammates to get mad. So they play better." Okay, so I lied a little. There was no such plan, obviously. I was just a bad goalie!

I played other sports, too. Soccer was important to me also. I wasn't as bad a goalie on the grass as I was on the ice. Baseball and football were also sports that occupied my interest, and I was talented at those sports. I also played a little basketball, but only for a short time in grade school. Soccer held on the longest, but eventually I felt that the game was more boring than fun.

My dad played football at Ohio State, though his career ended early because of a broken leg. His interest and athletic ability rubbed off on me and I became skilled at football. In the beginning I played flag football and then progressed to tackle football, and to be honest, I was pretty good at it.

I was enrolled at Shattuck–St. Mary's in Fairbault, Minnesota, for seventh and eighth grade. Shattuck–St. Mary's has a solid reputation for enrolling skilled hockey players who are destined for future stardom. My football interests ended while there because they would only allow students to play one sport. I was there to play hockey. That was my sport. And it was there that my dream to someday play professionally in the National Hockey League truly began.

Even though I advanced to the hockey school and that kind of took over my life, I have to go back some to talk about football for a second. I eventually transferred to Hill-Murray School in Maplewood, Minnesota, and they had no such restrictions on their student athletes, so I could play hockey *and* football. I think because of the success that my dad had at the college level, football was the first sport that I dreamed about playing at the professional level, and most certainly at the college level. Some sports were kind of boring for me and I never got into them much. But football? There was nothing boring about that.

As a youngster, I was really active. I was always around the other kids who loved sports. It didn't matter what the sport was. There were some kids who wanted to play and I was right there with them. I just simply loved to be moving. I've always had a close circle of friends, no matter where we have lived or what school I've been at, but I would have to say that my closest friends are my two cousins on my dad's side. Cannon is my age and Bo is a year younger. They are also talented hockey players. We have been close our entire lives.

I was once asked what my childhood was like. All I could think of was *sports, sports, sports, and more sports*, and *hockey, hockey, hockey, and more hockey*. Actually, though, I had a great childhood with many interests besides just sports. For instance, I loved to play golf—oops, back to sports again. I was also into movies quite a bit, too. Some of my all-time favorites are *Happy Gilmore*, *Slap*

Shot (there I am into hockey again), and *Shooter*. I have watched them all several times. I was never into the video game stuff like some kids are. Surprise, surprise: most of my video game action was centered around NHL-themed games. (Later, though, it was video games that occupied most of my time and got me through the endlessly long days in recuperation.)

For the most part, I had a pretty normal childhood. I'm kind of a history buff, I suppose. I remember spending a great deal of time watching the History Channel and Discovery Channel. I have always been interested in history, especially American history and events like the Boston Tea Party and other occurrences in our country's infancy. I think my mind is analytical in the right ways for history: I like to find out about things, go back to the past and see what happened. It might seem a kind of strange hobby for a kid, but it's true. It was definitely my favorite subject in school. I wasn't much of a reader, like my sister, so I got my history fix from the television and school. I was fascinated by it.

We first lived in Eagan, but when I began to have considerable success as a young hockey player at the Peewee level and in football, our family agreed that I would likely have a better chance to fully exploit those skills in the Edina school system. So we decided to move. I was the one who picked out the house. It had everything. For one thing, it was a rambler. Our previous house had a lot of stairs, which my dad didn't like, so it was made for him. It also had a pool. My sister, we joked, was some kind of fish, so the house was made for her, too. Everything about it seemed as if it was tailor-made for us. Initially our plan was to rent in the Edina school district, but when we found this house, we all liked it so much my parents purchased it. It is still our home today.

I was the one who found it. I searched online until I found the one that was just right for us. I don't know why, but early on in my life I developed this philosophy: if you want to get something done, do it yourself. *Get it done,* I taught myself.

Take this book, for instance. I had the book idea for quite some time after my medical issues took over my life. I remember trying to find an author. My dad and I had worked on getting it down for a while. We had a tape recorder and did some recording, but mostly, it just sat there and I got frustrated. We needed help. I used to ask my dad, "When are you going to find an author for my book? Is there anything new on the book?" Dad was working on it, I know he was, but I became impatient and decided to take matters into my own hands.

There were two people I knew who I thought might be able to assist me with this. One was Larry Hendrickson, the legendary hockey coach, and the other was Lou Nanne, former Minnesota North Stars player, coach, and executive. I knew that Mr. Nanne had two fairly recent books and had been on the book-signing circuit.

I found a way to get Mr. Nanne's phone number and I called him. I knew that he was aware of my medical history and my hockey abilities, though we had never formally met. I said, "Mr. Nanne, I have had this idea to write this book. My story. Can you help me to get an author?" He told me to contact the coauthor of his autobiography, *A Passion to Win.* And that's how I got in touch with Jim Bruton. Anything worth doing is worth doing yourself, as far as I'm concerned.

When we first moved to Edina, I knew it was going to be good for me because I could play a lot of sports there. Football was big for me in the upper-grade-school level. I played offense and defense. I was a middle linebacker on defense and scored a lot of touchdowns on offense as a running back. But there was a minor problem. There was a weight limit to be a running back and carry the football and I went over the weight limit. My dad helped out. I recall he got a motel room for us and we sat in a sauna until I was dying of thirst. I made the weight limit with about five pounds to spare and was cleared to play. My mom was not in favor of this method, and admittedly there was a period of time before she found out what we did. I don't think she was too happy about it.

I gave up a lot for hockey over the years, but it also broadened my horizons. I have also been able to travel extensively as a result—all over the state of Minnesota, and throughout the Midwest, Northeast, and Canada. I have stood in awe at Niagara Falls, and in a different sort of awe at Wayne Gretzky's restaurant in Toronto—which houses some of the legend's incredible memorabilia. I have been fortunate in my life to be blessed with some exceptional talent in sports. Years ago I had it all: a great family, wonderful friends, a future, and many dreams. And then all my hopes to play hockey in high school and perhaps in college and professionally came to a crashing end. My life, physically, would never be the same again. It wasn't one of those bumps in the road that people sometimes talk about; instead, it was a total change of course. Something that will have an effect on me and my family forever. But we are doing okay. We are moving on. We have struggled through it and it will never be over completely. Never. The early days were pretty tough—those days in the beginning, when all I could think about was, *What is happening to me?* I hate to think about how I could have recovered without them.

CHAPTER 2

Doctors and Denials

My life was firing on all cylinders. In my own private world of sports, everything had been going well for me. I can't think of a single thing that I would have wanted to be different. I lived and breathed sports. It was all I was interested in and all I wanted to do. It *consumed* me. Hockey was at the very top of the list—because I was really good at it and, more importantly, because I loved the sport, the arenas, the competition, and the speed of the game. It stimulated me. I was one of the best players on my Edina-area hockey team, and I was having a blast.

And then one day, something changed. This day, things just didn't seem right. I was in a hockey tournament in White Bear Lake, playing for our Peewee A-level team. Something was very wrong, but I didn't know what it was. I couldn't even explain it. At first I thought it was my skates that were the problem; they seemed to be really dull. I had taken a couple falls on the ice, which was very unusual for me. In fact, I rarely, if ever, fell during a game. When I went down a second time, I knew something was wrong. I was always in control of my body and my movements on the ice. For me, wearing skates was more comfortable than wearing shoes. If I could have been on them all the time, it would have been fine with me.

So what on earth was going on? It had to be the skate blades. They must be dull, I reasoned. It seemed to me the only explanation. I remember coming off the ice and taking off my skates. I was in a mild panic. I yelled to my dad, "My skates must be dull. My skates must be dull!" Dad quickly got them sharpened at the arena, and I went back out on the ice. But I kept falling. I would stumble and seemingly lose control of what I was doing. If it wasn't the skates, what was it? I didn't know, and it scared me.

Skating, handling the puck, moving up and down the ice was as natural for me as anything I ever did, and suddenly it seemed as if I had never done it before. For the first time in my life, it didn't come naturally. I had always been an aggressive hockey player—always around the puck, handling the puck, playing the game as it should be played. I was a good defenseman and rarely let anyone score when I was on the ice. On the offensive side, I had to work a little harder, but overall I held my own. I had a good shot and good puck control. I shot from my left side and worked hard at all aspects of the game I loved.

When I got the skates back, I thought the edge on my skate blades was gone completely. The arena sharpening hadn't worked—and the small sharpening tool that we carried had no effect either. My thoughts changed course. *If it's not the skate blades, then what is it? Is it me?* It's hard to describe, but it felt like everything my body knew about the game of hockey had disappeared. Everything that had come so naturally to me was out of reach. My reactions were slow. My confidence was shattered.

I had never had this feeling before. It shocked me. Suddenly all my skills seemed to disappear. My abilities, my confidence, my passion had gone in an instant. I didn't even have the excited feeling that I normally had when on the ice. Worse, I was scared.

I was playing as a defenseman during the game, but I had difficulty going forward and backward. This was new to me. I was trying to figure out exactly what I was doing wrong.

Meanwhile, something else was happening. I had a lot of pressure in my head. It was like that feeling you sometimes get on an airplane, when your ears get plugged and you feel like they are ready to pop at any second, but the pressure keeps building and building. My mind raced. I remembered that earlier in the season I played in a few games when a milder version of this occurred, but I had dismissed it.

There was another game, after which I came off the ice and told my mom, "Mom, there is really something wrong with me. We are going to have to figure out what it is, because I don't feel right out there on the ice. I don't know what it is but something is not right. I don't feel good at all." But then I was okay for a while so I quickly forgot about it—until it started happening again. The worst part was that I couldn't even explain what was happening because it was difficult to describe. All I knew was that I had lost my hockey skills, my ability to play the game the way I had been taught and the way I excelled at it.

The pressure was constant. My balance on the ice was terrible. And when I tried to go backward I would fall down. The best way I can describe it is that it felt like I had forgotten to take my skate guards off. That's the way it seemed to me at the time.

Everything about hockey had long been routine for me. It was comfortable. It was what I had done for years and years with no issues, no problems. I could do anything in my skates. I was so accustomed to wearing my skates that I could sense if the slightest thing was off—a blade was dull, a skate wasn't tight enough, that kind of thing. My skates were like an extension of my body.

At first, my mom thought it was some kind of a sinus problem because of the head pressure I was experiencing. After the game, she made an appointment for me to see an ear doctor first to find out what might be causing that pressure. Later, I had a CT scan, which identified the real problem. I call it a "ball of blood," but it is more commonly referred to as a brain bleed. The official name for what was discovered is cavernous hemangioma.

So we had a reason for the problem. It was a little more clear, but I wasn't willing to accept it at first. I remember coming out into the waiting room after the test and saying to my mom, "Come on, let's go. It's nothing. Let's go home. It's no big deal." I wanted out of there. I didn't want to hear any bad news.

My mom looked up at me and said, "Duke, sit down. I need to talk with you." I remember asking, "Wait, why do I need to sit down? Aren't we going home? What's wrong?" She was really quiet and said, "Duke, you need to sit down. I need to talk with you. There is something *seriously* wrong." I didn't want to hear it. I wanted no part of any bad news.

I didn't know what she was talking about. And frankly, I didn't want to know. I had just finished playing in a hockey tournament and felt halfway fine again—I mean, nothing serious. I felt like whatever I had experienced was no big deal. Sure, I was having some problems on the ice that were concerning to me, no question about that, but something seriously wrong? No way! I had a lot more hockey to play, and I was not going to let a problem in one game derail me from what was ahead.

My mom didn't get into the details of what had been found on the test, but she kept clearly saying to me that there was a serious problem that had been discovered. We ended up leaving the clinic where I had the test and driving directly to the hospital. I still had not been told what exactly was wrong. All I knew was we were on the way to the hospital for more tests. *Tests? Why do I need more tests? I'm okay. There is nothing wrong, everything is fine*, I remember thinking. I knew it. At least I think I did. I suppose I was in denial.

I was admitted into the hospital and they began to run a series of tests on me. Even so, I wasn't concerned. I figured it was just some kind of minor setback. During the night, the medical staff checked on me seemingly constantly because I had a low heart rate and they suspected that something might be wrong. But the low rate was caused by the good condition my body was in from being an athlete, nothing more. It made me feel good to know that I was in great shape; it was a little consolation considering the position I was in at the time.

My memory is a little foggy looking back, but as far as I can remember, I was told I had a condition in my brain stem that at that point was inoperable. The doctor told us that it would likely return with greater severity in about two years, but apparently there was nothing that could be done until then. (As it happens, that first doctor was right on the money with his estimate.)

Even though I had been discharged, it took about two months for most of the symptoms to clear up. I was out of sports during that period of time, and it was really tough for me because so much of my identity was wrapped up in that. Worse, I was in bed most of the time. I couldn't do much at all. I hung out with some of my friends from Edina who'd come over, but mostly I just lay around. It was torture for someone like me who was used to keeping active all day. My grandpa—my mom's dad—would come over and stay with me from time to time, and we would build model airplanes together.

Meanwhile, my Peewee team was playing without me. They were out there on the ice playing the game I loved, and I was lying around the house doing nothing. It drove me crazy. It wasn't right. I should have been out there playing alongside my hockey buddies. I looked forward to every part of the hockey experience: the anticipation of the game, going to the arena, putting on my uniform and my skates, chasing the puck during warm-ups, shooting...there wasn't a part of it that I didn't love, and being away from it was difficult—especially knowing that they could go on without me.

During this period, I was home virtually all the time. Our Edina house was not yet in order because we had just moved in. Everything was in total disarray. Most of our possessions were still in boxes. I was staying in my parents' room, and all around me was chaos. It wasn't a new home, but we were in the midst of some fairly major remodeling.

It was a tough time for all of us. I was the one who picked out the house for us, and then while everything was going on to get the house in shape for us, I was stuck in bed most of the time. I felt helpless. Never in my wildest dreams could I have imagined something like this happening to me.

My Peewee team finished third in the state tournament—and I missed it. I missed all the games, all the excitement, all the enjoyment. I took it hard. Even with all my health issues, I was mostly upset over what I had lost in hockey. I ached inside.

Those days it seemed as if my parents were taking me to different doctors every day. We sought opinions from all kinds of different doctors to be sure the initial diagnosis was correct. Through it all we kind of stuck with the original opinion of Dr. Nahib. Most of the doctors we saw did not want to be involved with my case because it was "too risky"—at least that's what I was told. Dr. Nahib was the only one who was willing to take on my problem.

During the two months of my initial recuperation, very little happened. It was close to Easter and I was feeling a little better. The doctor told me that once I felt up to it, I should go and do what I wanted to do. "Go live your life," he encouraged me. His plan was to keep tabs on what was happening and deal with any problems as they developed. In the meantime, he wanted for me to do what kids do at my age and enjoy my life. I had two years, he predicted, before those problems would likely recur, at which point we would deal with it together.

As the spring went on, I started to feel really good again. Even though we had moved to Edina and could have gotten into the Edina system for athletics, my dad thought that I should go to Shattuck–St. Mary's, a private boarding school in Fairbault, Minnesota—to play hockey. I think he felt that I had some outstanding skills as a young player, and he knew the reputation of Shattuck–St. Mary's.

Of course, Shattuck–St. Mary's is well-known locally—and nationally—as a breeding ground for young, highly skilled hockey players. Wayne Gretzky's kid went to Shattuck. Sidney Crosby went to Shattuck. So you see what I mean. If you were accepted there and were a hockey player, you had to be pretty good, period.

J.P. Parise, a former Minnesota North Stars player, was a scout for Shattuck and he was aware of my play. I had practiced there earlier, and even though I didn't perform very well, J.P. told my dad that he had seen something in me that let him know I was going to be a good player; his instincts and all of his experience apparently told him that. He told my dad something to the effect that he thought I had a lot of promise and a bright future. J.P. had come to a lot of my games and saw me quite often. Eventually, I was given the nod to enroll at Shattuck to play hockey. I entered in the seventh grade and stayed for the next two years.

I feel that I was destined to go there, and I began my hockey career again with fresh hope for the future. Shattuck–St. Mary's had six teams all playing at different levels. I was on the Bantam Tier I team. It was near the bottom, but I wasn't discouraged; everyone starts in the Bantam tier there. It was also the top Bantam team there, and I was playing some ninth-graders even though I was in the seventh grade.

The first year I didn't like the dorms, so I stayed with my grandparents, my dad's parents. They got a condo right near the campus so I could stay with them. It wasn't the only reason for their move, but it was one of them. It was great for me because I was living in comfortable surroundings and I really got to know my grandparents well, especially my grandpa. There was also a golf course nearby, and the two of us went to the course often over those two years.

Hockey was going very well. I was in the seventh grade playing with older kids, so it wasn't all roses. The game changed for me. The coaching was different and there was a huge learning curve. I was doing well, but I did have a hard time scoring goals. But I was hanging in there on defense; rarely did the opposition score when I was on the ice. Overall, I was holding my own.

One of the main reasons I loved playing at Shattuck–St. Mary's was because of my coach, Murray Eaves. Coach Eaves had played college hockey at the University of Michigan and was an outstanding player. Because he went to Michigan and my dad went to Ohio State, to this day they give each other the business because of the rivalry between the schools.

Mr. Eaves left after his sophomore year at UM, after being drafted in the third round by the Winnipeg Jets. He was with the Winnipeg organization for six years and then was traded to the Edmonton Oilers, where he spent another season. He played a total of 57 games in the National Hockey League as a center. He played a few years in Europe before returning to coach in the Detroit Red Wings organization at the minor league level. He became a head coach at what would be considered about the AA level.

Later, after an interview with Parise, he was hired to coach hockey at Shattuck. Coach Eaves has been an important part of my life and has had great influence on me throughout the years.

While at Shattuck, our team traveled a lot. I saw a lot of the country in those years. I learned to be disciplined and do things on my own. It was a lot of work, but I enjoyed it. Our team was very good and we accomplished a third-place finish in the national championships; that was very special for me and for our team.

I never had the captain *C* on my jersey, but I always felt that I was one of the team leaders. I also made some good friends. In our second year we got fifth place in the national championships, and although we did not do as well, I was pleased with our status and overall accomplishments. I felt like I was playing well.

As far as my medical issues went, I forgot about them. It was out of sight, out of mind. And I didn't even have a blip of a recurrence during that time. I was feeling great. I was living in the moment. And everything was good. Dr. Nahib's "two year" prediction didn't ever creep up on me; I had forgotten about it completely.

I played with a lot of good players and got a lot of experience. I also played golf at Shattuck and really enjoyed it. I was nothing special on the links, but it kept me busy when hockey—year-round at Shattuck—didn't.

After my second year, I felt like my time at Shattuck was over. The competition was fierce; I competed with some of the best-known names in youth hockey. But I didn't like that, because I always felt that the bigger the name, the bigger the family connections, the more attention that was paid to those individuals. At times, that was difficult for me to accept. But the bigger reason to leave Shattuck was football. I really missed playing football, and I couldn't do both at Shattuck. So I transferred to Hill-Murray for the ninth grade.

I could have gone to Edina, where we were living, because their programs in football and hockey were also very good. But I had my mind set on Hill-Murray because I knew some kids who had been at Shattuck who were there. Hill-Murray was also the reigning state champion in hockey and was well-known as a great hockey school. Furthermore, we had family connections. My uncle on my mom's side went to Hill-Murray.

Maybe the biggest reason I wanted to go to Hill-Murray, though, was their hockey coach, Bill Lechner. He has been a real credit to the hockey world and to young people. He was an exceptional athlete in his own right at Cretin High School and then at the University of St. Thomas, excelling especially in baseball and hockey. Besides being the head hockey coach, he is also Hill-Murray's athletic director, overseeing 24 varsity sports for boys and girls. He is also the school's longtime baseball coach. Under Coach Lechner's leadership Hill-Murray hockey has won three state championships, and his overall hockey coaching record is closing in on 300 wins. Furthermore, he has a sterling reputation as a super nice guy.

Because of all this, I set my sights on Hill-Murray. I wanted Coach Lechner to give me a chance to play varsity as a ninth-grader. (The Edina coach was not willing to do that, by contrast.) I would have to go through tryouts—along with everybody else on the team, including the returning varsity players—but Coach Lechner told me that if I was good enough I could make the varsity squad as a freshman.

Coming in as a ninth-grader, I realized how good this team was. After all, they were defending state champions! Coach Lechner expected a lot and it was tough. I was small compared to the older kids. Older made a big difference. They were bigger, stronger, and had a lot of experience I didn't have. Every day's practice was, for the most part, a tryout session.

Coach Schafhauser was the defensive coach, and he completely changed the game for me. He played hockey at Hill-Murray from 1987 to 1989 and then played collegiate hockey at Boston College. After college, he played professionally in Europe for five years in Switzerland before his career abruptly ended. He was seriously injured in a game when he was checked in the back and went headfirst into the boards. He incurred a spinal cord injury, which resulted in permanent paralysis.

Later, Coach Lechner invited him back to coach the junior varsity, and for the past 17 seasons he has been the assistant varsity coach, focusing on the defensemen. We had a great relationship and I have a great deal of respect for him. I mean, he coaches in a wheelchair and does an exceptional job. He is inspiring in so many ways.

Leading up to the regular season, the varsity team traveled some around the state—and I gave it my all every moment I was on the ice. I *had* to give it everything I had to stay with these older kids. It was my dream, no doubt, and I was doing okay. And the best part was I was feeling good. My medical problems were a distant memory. I was excelling at the sport that I loved and had a chance to make the varsity team at Hill-Murray. I had put my past difficulties completely out of my mind.

CHAPTER 3

The Puck Drops

Ninth grade. Hill-Murray. I was living the good life. I had played on the ninth-grade football team that fall—at running back and defensive end. We weren't very good—in fact, we lost every game—but I met a lot of kids, made some good friends, and was really enjoying my new school.

The hockey tryouts had been weighing heavily on my mind for some time. I had been preparing mentally and physically for an all-out effort to make varsity. The tryouts ran over the course of a full week, and I put everything I had out on the ice. After the first few tryout days, I was so tired that I felt like I could hardly move, and I made some really dumb mistakes. I couldn't believe some of the things I was doing. I was failing at the basics, as far as I was concerned. I missed passes, fumbled around with the puck, skated slowly, messed up shots—they were not a good few days for me.

I was not very happy with myself, but kept at it and didn't get discouraged. I didn't know what to expect but suspected I had probably played my way off the varsity squad. When the coach posted the list of those who made the team, I hung back. I didn't want to see it because I was afraid of being disappointed.

Those who didn't make the varsity team would play on the junior varsity—and I was not looking forward to that. I went to Hill-Murray to make the varsity, but I knew as only a ninth-grader it would be very difficult to achieve that goal. My friend J.D. Cotroneo went up to look at the list and came running up to me. He said, "Duke! Duke! You are on the team! You made it!" I didn't believe him and told him so. "No, no, Duke, honest, you made the team. You're on the team!" I was in shock. Chills ran up and down my spine.

I still wasn't sure what to think. Had I played better than I thought? Was I too critical of myself? Did the coaches see something in me that I missed? Was it really true that I had made the varsity squad at Hill-Murray School, the defending Minnesota state hockey champs?

I waited until the players dispersed, and then meandered over to take a look for myself. There it was: Duke Pieper. My name was on the list. I didn't show any outward emotion, but inside I was ecstatic. I felt fantastic. My guts were churning and I had goose bumps—goose bumps! Butterflies fluttered in my stomach. I was thrilled! I had made the Hill-Murray varsity as a ninth-grader, a freshman. It was unbelievable! I kept the news to myself and didn't celebrate with anyone else.

My dad was waiting outside in the car for me, as he had every day after tryouts. I got in the car and he immediately asked, "Well, what team did you make?" I told him, "I made the varsity," and he gave me a big hug. His face was wrought with joy and I even saw a few tears in his eyes. The look on his face made it all worthwhile. I will never forget it.

That night I had to go and get all my equipment because we were leaving the next day for a scrimmage in Grand Rapids. It had been quite a day. I was reeling from the pressure of the week, the tryouts, disappointment in my poor performance, and then exuberance at finding out the results. There was no doubt, I was living the good life.

The next morning we got on the bus. The new players—including me!—were sitting at the front of the bus and the older players were at the back. The older guys called the young players to the back one by one, and from that moment on we were a part of the team.

We played several scrimmages, and I think I did okay. One thing I found out was that playing with older kids was in some ways easier than I had anticipated. We had an exceptional team and it seemed like all I really had to do was pass the puck up the ice to the forwards and they would do the rest. As a defenseman, I had always been comfortable with that aspect of the game. I could protect our net, get the puck out of our zone, and handle my responsibilities.

After those first few scrimmages it was clear that our team was firing on all cylinders. We were playing really well as a team, and I was looking forward to the regular season beginning.

If you had asked me then, I would have said that everything was perfect. Everything had gone exactly as I'd hoped, almost as if it were scripted: I had transferred to Hill-Murray, made the varsity team, and was holding my own on the ice with players much older than me. The future was bright and I couldn't wait to get there.

On the morning of our first game I woke up feeling a little bit different, a bit off. I had been wearing a new necklace; maybe that was the culprit, I reasoned. That sounds a little bizarre, perhaps, but there had to be something. I got out of bed and walked down the hall to the bathroom, thinking that something was not right. By the time I got to school I was definitely not feeling very well. I still thought it might be the necklace. I told one of my friends that morning, "Yeah, man, this necklace is super weird." I gave it to my friend. "Keep it. I don't want it," I told him.

I didn't know what was up. It wasn't like my eyes were bad or my balance was off. There was nothing that I could really put my finger on; I just knew that something in me was not right. It was almost like things were not aligned right. Something was out of whack. I started to become troubled by the feeling. Even so, I never gave a single thought to my brain issue or Dr. Nahib's prediction. *Never*.

Over the course of the past couple years my dad would occasionally ask if I was experiencing any problems and I would always say the same thing. "Why are you even bringing this up? I am having no issues at all. None," I'd fire back. I didn't even want to think about it.

It might seem rather odd that I never gave the whole medical thing much of my attention, but I had good reason. I mean, why would I want to concern myself with worrying about it until something actually happened? No possible good can come from that kind of thinking, just waiting for the puck to drop. So why would I want to put myself in that kind of position? It made no sense to me, and I was going to have no part of it. Some part of me deep down knew that day would come, but I hadn't spent any time thinking of it, so it didn't immediately occur to me that my brain might be the problem.

So all that day, I was convinced that I was feeling lousy because of that rotten necklace. I was glad I gave it away, but it didn't help. I still had this funny feeling. I went through the motions of my day, classes, lunch, more classes. I tried to dismiss the eerie feeling and put it in the back of my mind. After all, we were play-ing our first game that night. I was pumped up! My mind needed to be on the game, not some ridiculous feeling that I couldn't even explain to myself, let alone anyone else.

Aboard the bus on the way to the game I was listening to some music. I was thinking about how weird I felt. *Why now? Why tonight, before our first game?*

Our game was at Burnsville High School. They were ranked high—third in the state, I think—and we were ranked No. 1. So it was a big game for us to open the season with, and even more so for me, because it was my first game as a player on the varsity. I needed to play my best and prove to myself and others that I deserved to be on the varsity team.

Everything about hockey at this level was new to me. I was curious about it all—the environment, the arena, their team, our team…all the things that one would expect for a first game with a new team. I was a little nervous, that was expected, but I had played in some big games in the past at Shattuck and had always handled pressure quite well.

We got in the locker room and everything was so exciting and new to me. I had played a lot of hockey games in my life, but this was something really special. I was about to embark on my first game as a freshman on a state championship hockey team!

I always got fired up for games. I really took it all in and appre-ciated all that came with playing hockey. I loved to watch the fans, play before a big crowd. And this would be the biggest crowd I'd played for yet, no question about that.

At Shattuck–St. Mary's the crowds were never that big because our team was made up of players from all over the world. But this night, our first game, opening night was different. These were local boys, in front of a hometown crowd, playing the defending state champions. I was bright-eyed as I scanned the arena—the crowd, our opponents, and then my teammates. I couldn't wait to get onto the ice, my element.

My dad and uncle were in the stands at the game, while my mom and other relatives were at home watching the game on television. The game was being covered by one of our local channels. It was big-time.

We went out for some preliminary warm-ups, did a little running and calisthenics. Despite the adrenaline I felt surging inside me, something was not right. My past medical difficulties had been pushed out of my mind for such a long time that even as my memory dredged up the possibility, I was not about to jump to that conclusion. Still, that little voice lingered. *This can't be the same as before, can it? Was the doctor right? Is my brain bleed returning?*

After we finished the calisthenics, I began to realize that I might not be able to play in the game. We went out on the ice for our pregame warm-ups, and I noticed the size of the crowd. It was big, and they were not on our side. As if to echo my thought, the visitors let us know. All these Burnsville fans began really chirping at us.

At one point during warm-ups, I was skating toward the goal… and it didn't look right to me. It was *off*. I had played a lot of hockey by this point in my life and my instincts were sharp. Was it me or was it the goal? I didn't tell anyone. I mean, how could I explain it? "The goal looks off. The net looks off." Come on, who would listen to that nonsense?

I kept skating around and took a shot at the net and then I really noticed something. The net, my stick, the way the puck came off my stick—everything about that moment was different.

Nothing felt right. I kept on skating around trying to shake the feeling. I was one of the last players on our team to get off the ice to go back to the locker room. I knew I was in trouble.

When we got to the locker room, the team was getting assembled to listen to the coach's pregame speech. I went to Coach Lechner and said, "Coach, this is not going to happen for me tonight." He looked at me and said, "What are you talking about?" I told him, "Coach, I don't think I should play in the game." Coach Lechner looked at me and said, "Duke, it's just nerves. You're nervous. You'll be all right." What he said was understandable. After all, I was only in the ninth grade, playing my very first varsity game. Of course I was nervous! Except it wasn't nerves. I knew that.

The coach felt that because I had never been in this kind of setting, it was all new to me, I was experiencing what a lot of kids feel before their first game. Of course, he didn't know a thing about my medical history, not that I would have acknowledged that as a possibility. But I certainly knew that it wasn't nerves. I wasn't a nervous guy. I had played in some pretty big games for Shattuck–St. Mary's—we had competed in the nationals and played some incredible big-time games. The pressure of the big game never bothered me. I was one of the steady ones.

In that moment, I just knew that I didn't want to screw something up for the team. I didn't want to go out on the ice and hurt our team's chances to win the game. It was our first game and we were playing against a top opponent, so it was all the more important that we come away with a victory.

"Coach, please listen," I told him. "If I go out there I am going to really mess something up, and I don't want to do that. You have got to trust me on this." So Coach Lechner told me to go talk to the trainer about what was going on with me. After a little more discussion, Coach Lechner realized that it was important to take precautions and accepted the fact that I would not play in the game. He knew it was important to get me checked out. Like me, he thought it was just a brief radar blip and that I would be back the next day or so.

The trainer came over and looked at me, but I knew right from the start that she was not going to be able to tell me anything. There was no way that she was going to know what was wrong with me when I couldn't even describe it myself. *I* didn't even know. What I did know, however, was I could not play in the game.

I ended up taking off my gear. I felt so alone. My dream was unraveling. The rest of the team was listening to the coach talk and were getting ready to go out on the ice and start the game—without me. The feeling I was having at this point was unexplainable. It was unbearable agony.

Here, right in front of me was my dream, something that I had worked so hard for. I should have been up in the front listening to the coach, getting ready to play my first varsity game with a state champion team, and I was taking off my gear in the back of the room. It was one of the worst moments of my life.

Still, in my mind, I thought it was only a slight setback. I didn't realize at the time what was happening. I thought I would get checked out and be back on the ice the next day. I was wrong, because there would be more coming. I would never go out on the ice with my team again.

If I had realized at the time it would be my last game, I probably would have done everything possible to play. I mean if it was going to be my last game, why not go out and play? I think those would have been my thoughts as I look back. This is what initially comes into my mind, but then as I stop and look at what I am really about,

I would have to say that I would have taken my skates off anyway. I say that because it would have been too selfish to go on the ice when I knew I would be hurting my team.

The entire day and that special night will always remain somewhat of a blur. It was so unsettling, the entire day, I mean. When I was skating on the ice during a game or during warm-ups, I could tell if the littlest thing was wrong. I knew if my skate blades were a little dull. I knew if my stick wasn't taped quite right. I knew if my pads were a little off, if my jersey wasn't tucked in, if my laces were too tight or too lose. Hockey was so natural to me. It came so easy and was such a huge part of my life.

Given all this, obviously coming off the ice after warm-ups, I knew there was something seriously wrong and that I was not going to be able to play in the game. There was no way I could play. Everything seemed wrong: my skating, my shooting, the way the net looked, the way the puck came off my stick, just everything.

I knew if I decided to go back out there anyway, there was absolutely no chance of me playing well. I knew the game was going to be on local television and I was convinced that I would hurt the team and embarrass myself. I mean this was the first game of the regular season, my first game, and I did not want to play badly. It was all too important. I have to be honest when I say that the game, my future, my relationship with the coaches and my teammates was all too important to me to jeopardize. There was just no way I was going to play.

My only option was to go in and tell the coach what was happening and take off my gear. *Just a hiccup*, I thought to myself. *Go in, take off my gear, get fixed what needs fixing, and return to the team and prepare for the next game.* That was my thought process. Nothing more serious than that.

Even though I wasn't worried about my health, leaving the game was extremely disappointing. In fact, coming off the ice before my first varsity game was as tough a time as anything I had experienced to that point in my life. When I went into the locker room, I knew what I had to do. I went to my side of the locker room and began to take my skates off. The room was kind of divided: one set of benches on one side of a wall and another set on the other side. My side was for the defensemen and the goalies. Meanwhile, everyone else had gone to the other side to listen to the coach give the pregame talk. So I was alone for the most part. There were a couple guys around who were not going to play who drifted in, but that was it. Then again, I suppose there could have been a hundred people in the room and I still would have felt alone.

The room was kind of a tan color—not a great place, just a nondescript place to get dressed for the game. There weren't really lockers to use, so everyone's gear and clothing was piled on the benches and the floor. I could hear the coach and the team on the other side of the room, getting set to go out on the ice.

My mind was spinning. I remember being surprised that no one really asked me what I was doing. Why was I taking off my skates and all my hockey gear? What was I doing? One guy asked if I was okay and I mumbled back that I was fine. If I had explained what was going on, it would not have been much of an explanation—because I honestly didn't know *what* was happening. All I knew was things were not right for me and hadn't been right all day. The coach thought I was just nervous, but I knew there was something more to it.

Sitting there alone in that locker room was not one of my best moments. I sat by myself while the coach talked to the team and I was alone when the team left the locker room for the ice. I was upset and confused. Yet it never crossed my mind that I was having a recurrence of my brain issue. Even when I was out on the ice and really struggling, I never thought about what that doctor had told me. There were too many other things going on. It was my first high school hockey game. The arena was full of fans. The home fans were yelling at us. There was a lot of excitement. I was trying to get myself in some kind of shape to be able to play. It was an exciting time and I was filled with emotions.

As I look back, it all seems so ridiculous. I have this problem. I don't know what it is and I cannot explain it. Try telling someone *that*. I didn't even know how to say it. *"Coach, I can't play today because something is not right."*

To which the coach would respond, *"What do you mean something is not right?"*

"I don't know, something is not right. I can't explain it. I don't feel right, but I don't know how to be any more specific than that." I guess it is easy to figure out why I didn't tell anyone.

I have thought about this a great deal over the years. What did I feel like that night? It was not like a headache, when you can say, "My head hurts." It was not like the flu, when you can say, "I have a fever, aches, and nausea." It wasn't like a pulled muscle, when you can say, "It's right here in my left hamstring." It wasn't like any of those things—but after a lot of thought I have developed somewhat of an explanation.

It was like everything was tilted for me that whole day. When I got up in the morning at home and went to the bathroom, I recall thinking, *Whoa, what is wrong here?* The same thing can be said about the ice during pregame warm-ups. Everything I did that day was abnormal and confusing.

I also liken it to being on an airplane. My head felt funny. I had that type of feeling when at times you feel a little off because of the pressure buildup—at least I have that feeling sometimes when I fly. I simply felt a little weird, as if my balance was off. It is hard to explain. There was no physical pain; things were just different. If I were tested on being able to describe exactly how I felt, I would fail miserably because this is my only explanation, the best I can do to describe it.

As I undid my skates, I was in a daze. Maybe I was in some kind of denial. Maybe in the back of my mind I really did know that the problem was much more serious than I was letting on. I say this because when I talked to my mom on the phone I told her that there was something seriously wrong with me. I guess I did know but was unable to accept it. When I left the ice after warm-ups, I suppose I *knew* but obviously was in denial. I was one of the last players to leave the ice; I guess I wanted to be sure. I wanted to be absolutely convinced that I could not play in the game. I was. I knew.

If I had accepted at the time that this was going to be the end, I would have been totally devastated. Maybe I would have done something stupid, like gone out there and attempted to play for the last time. I don't like to think about it because it is not me; I would not have wanted to hurt my team.

I took all my gear off and went out to try to find my dad. I looked everywhere but could not find him. I was so anxious. I didn't know what to think. What was happening to me?

I went outside and still could not find him. I tried his cell phone but he didn't answer. Considering all the noise in the arena, it wasn't surprising. But I was getting increasingly troubled. So I called my mom. I didn't want to do that because I was afraid she would freak out. She is the type to get really excited about things, and I was worried that she would be really upset and scared.

I told her, "Mom, I need you to sit down so I can talk to you." I said, "Mom, I think it has come back. You know, my brain issue. I think it has come back." As much as I did not want to believe it, I guess I knew. And I think she knew it too, once I told her what had happened.

A couple years previous, I had asked my doctor, "How will I know if this problem is returning? What will happen? What will I be experiencing to know that it's back?"

The doctor said, "You will know. Trust me, you will know." That didn't really help much at the time—and it probably contributed somewhat to why I had just put it out of my mind for those two years. I didn't worry about it. I wasn't looking for certain things to occur because there were no certain symptoms to look out for. All I had to go on was "You'll know." And in that moment, outside the arena, I began to understand. As much as I didn't want it to be, it was.

Between the time I told my coach that I couldn't play and the time I spoke with my mom, I believe that I began to realize what was happening to me. But I pushed those thoughts to the back burner as much as I could. Even as I became more and more convinced, I kept shutting the thought down. *No way! Not now! Forget it!* I tried my best to block it out of my mind because I did not want to believe it.

I was eventually able to get in contact with my uncle Dave in the stands and he told me where to find Dad. Once we finally connected, I told him, "Dad, we have to go home. We need to get an MRI or something because things are not right with me." Dad is calm with things. He knows how to handle tough times. We left the game and went home. There, we discussed what was occurring with me in detail before heading to the emergency room. For a few minutes before we went to the hospital, I watched the game on television. It wasn't any fun to watch. In fact, it was really difficult for me to see. I should have been there.

We went to the emergency room—and they sent me home. This convinced me even more that it was only a minor setback and that there would be a quick fix. Obviously, it didn't turn out that way.

CHAPTER 4

Hospitals and Heartaches

The emergency room doctors looked me over...and summarily turned us away. They sent us home. But we knew for sure at that point that it was happening again; my brain issues had resurfaced. So we made an appointment with the neurologist.

We had an MRI scheduled and the doctor was to give us the results. After the MRI, we sat in the waiting room, agonizing over the results. Every minute felt like hours. When the doctor finally appeared, he told us that I needed surgery.

I remember crying once I heard the news. I was scared. I didn't know what to think. I also don't like needles, so the thought of surgery, needles, and whatever other torturous things they were going to do to me really tore me up. I don't remember what I was told about the procedure. But if I had needed ankle surgery, it would have disturbed me just as much. At the time I didn't even know the severity of my condition—that I had a 5 percent chance of living. Those are not good odds. Not having the opportunity to be on the ice with my teammates was disappointing, but it was a far cry from wondering if I was going to live or die.

The whole thing was devastating. I can remember crying my eyes out—and we were not even at the hospital yet. Maybe it was my squeamishness, or maybe it was self-preservation, but I didn't want to know any of the details of the procedure. *Let's just do the surgery and leave the facts and details to someone else, thank you very much.* I knew my parents could deal with that.

I'm not sure why, but we had a couple days before I would have the surgery. While waiting, I stayed at home and played video games—*Call of Duty*, I think, was what I spent most of my time doing. I tried not to think about what I was facing. I concentrated on the video games and that was all. During this time, I did not have much contact with anyone outside my immediate family. I didn't know too many people at Hill-Murray, since I was still new there, and frankly I'm not sure who knew about my issues.

All this time, I had never expected to be there, on the precipice of major surgery. I never thought my condition would come back, much less threaten my life. In short, I did not realize the full impact that this was having or was going to have on me.

Staring down major surgery, one would think that any kid going through such a thing would be totally troubled by what he or she would be facing. I didn't feel that way at all because I was in complete denial. I was totally immersed in keeping my mind off the problem. Totally. I exerted all my energy toward this singular goal, and the video games got me through it.

My mom handled it all much better than I anticipated she would. Like my dad, she was calm when I first told her. And she quickly became the one who handled everything. What was happening was not good—not good at all. The odds were certainly not in my favor.

(Someone later told me—I can't recall whom it was—that I may be the only person who ever survived this type of brain lesion.)

At the time prior to the surgery, I knew nothing about the reality of what I would soon be facing. I did not ask because I did not want to know. That crazy, unexplainable physical feeling remained. I was not myself. I felt exactly the same as I had when I came off the ice. I was in trouble, very serious trouble. But I was in denial. And maybe, as I look back, that was a good thing.

I have very little recollection of what happened next. My best way to recall the events and make an attempt to explain what happened is to reference the website that my family set up for my family, friends, and other loved ones. It initially read:

Duke had a cavernous hemangioma in his brain stem. (I like to refer to it as a ball of blood.)

On December 2, 2008, Duke had a reoccurrence of symptoms that are the result of the cavernous hemangioma putting pressure on his brain stem nerves. After further tests we understood that the CH had doubled in size and bled. On Friday, December 5, 2008, we were told that Duke required surgery to remove the CH from his brain stem. The area of the brain stem where the surgery will be done houses the cranial nerves. At this point we were aware that Duke may experience further complications with his eyes, facial features, swallowing function, breathing, and heart function, and have balance issues along with several other areas.

On Saturday, December 6, 2008, he was admitted to Abbott Northwestern Hospital to the ICU (Intensive Care Unit) awaiting surgery scheduled for Monday morning, December 8, 2008. Duke had begun a steroid treatment on Friday that would continue throughout the surgery and post-operation time to keep the swelling down in the brain.

Duke had a long day on Monday. He began his journey at 5:30 AM with an MRI. At 7:45 AM surgery began. His family was at the hospital with him for support and prayer. At 3:45 PM Duke's neurosurgeon spoke with the family regarding the surgery. The MRI picture showed that they were able to remove all of the CH successfully from the brain stem. Duke remained in recovery until about 6:00 PM and then he was brought up to the Neuro ICU. Duke remained on a ventilator for the evening and into the next day. Tuesday afternoon they took Duke off the ventilator and his recovery journey began.

During the next 48 hours, neurologically Duke was recovering very well. He was viewed as a miracle child. One of the complications that we were seeing at the time was hallucinations and disorientation during the evenings and eventually beginning to occur during the daytime as well. With the progress Duke was making neurologically, by Friday, December 12, Duke was moved to the eighth floor and out of the ICU.

His complications continued to worsen and overtake the short-term success Duke had accomplished. Sunday evening Duke was brought back to the ICU and several tests were run to get a better grasp on his current state. A spinal tap, CT, and blood work began on Sunday night, December 14, 2008. Duke began antibiotics Sunday for meningitis, which doctors were working to rule out. At this point Duke had multiple complications and several doctors were consulted. Duke was finally taken off steroids because doctors felt they may be contributing to his condition.

During the week of December 15, doctors continued to

work on what could be the cause of Duke's worsening condition. On Wednesday Duke had an MRI, spinal tap, and several other tests to monitor progress. At this point he has had no food and little sleep. Late in the week, it appeared that Duke's antibiotics began to work and we were seeing progress in Duke's condition.

On Tuesday, December 23, 2008, Duke was still in the Neuro ICU and his fever spiked to 103 degrees, along with other complications. Doctors and nurses monitored him through Christmas Eve and Christmas Day taking blood cultures, and on Friday Duke had another spinal tap and head CT. The spinal tap results showed abnormalities in the spinal fluid and new antibiotics were started. The CT showed no change, which was good. Additional blood cultures, X-rays, and testing began.

On December 28, 2008, we are still in the ICU and hoping the antibiotics take effect. Duke has not eaten and has lost a lot of weight, which has resulted in him being very weak. Our next step is for Duke to have a swallow test to make sure he is not aspirating. Our hope is to get food into his system for strength. A g-tube may need to be installed.

This was the first thing written on my Caring Bridge website, which my family maintained to keep everyone updated on my condition, and it is still amazing to me every time I take a look at it. For one thing, I don't remember any of this happening to me in those first uneasy days. The many, many further entries written by family and friends down the road have been incredible. When I read some of them, in many ways I still find it hard to believe all of this actually happened to me. In some ways, it is like a dream, or maybe better said, a living nightmare.

One entry on the site, from December 24, 2008, came from a friend, and it gives me chills when I read it. Because I always try to keep a positive outlook, I try to stay away from these kinds of things most of the time, but it gives a good perspective of what was going on at the time. It reads in part:

> To all Duke's supporters, I am writing this email to everyone whom I know that has come in contact with Duke Pieper.
>
> I just got off the phone with Mark, Duke's dad, regarding an update on Duke's condition. For those of you who are not aware, Duke underwent major surgery on his brain a few weeks ago. He battled hard and was starting to rebound. Duke then went into a coma and had a number of doctors treating him for an infection. Duke came out of the coma late last week. Mark was thrilled. He said he knows the road to recovery will be long, but I will take that over the alternative. Mark and his family have been extremely busy as we could all imagine, and he has been keeping me updated every four or five days. I told him we would relay the information to everyone we knew.
>
> Today was not a great update...
>
> Duke is very weak and in a tremendous amount of pain. Mark said that every step forward comes with two steps back. They can't give him painkillers because it will impact their data. He can't sit up for fear the blood will rush to the brain. He has a high fever and has trouble even talking.
>
> He has told his dad that he "just wants to die." The doctors initially thought if all had gone well Duke would have been walking 10 days after the surgery. It has now been three weeks. Mark and his family have not given up hope!!!!

The website provides a good summary of everything I went through, the many ups and downs. It illustrates, as my dad has often said, that just as things were going well with one step ahead, there would be two steps in reverse. One such entry came on March 18, 2009. I had actually come home and had been doing well for a period of time, and then:

Duke had a very difficult night prior to surgery. He had another MRI this morning, several X-rays, and blood draws. He was experiencing extreme pain that seemed unbearable and unmanageable to the medical staff. Liz and Mark have been at Gillette Children's Hospital and are now back at Abbott Northwestern again, tending to Duke around the clock. This surgery is no exception.

Duke came through the surgery according to doctors. Doctors feel like they have cleaned out the infection. Draws from the infected area will be cultured to help diagnose and treat his current infection. Duke's doctor is not certain what is causing the pain.

Duke has high blood pressure and some complications with his heart that are being reviewed and monitored. He is back in the ICU tonight, after his two-and-a-half-hour surgery today.

Duke is predicted to have a longer recovery than experienced with his last infection surgery, but we will know more in the next few days. Several medications have been necessary to treat Duke's anxiety regarding his status and to treat the pain he is experiencing.

Liz and Mark are troubled by his current situation. Duke's condition is rare and complicated. Doctors are working to overcome this current setback so that Duke can get back to Gillette and continue rehabilitation—moving in the right direction.

Indeed, there was a time in there when I wanted to know all there was to know about dying, and for a brief period thought that would be the better solution to all these endless goings-on. It was also a real possibility. On two occasions, my parents actually began planning my funeral. That's how close I was to death.

The condition is called a cavernous hemangioma, though it is a lot easier to just call it a brain bleed. The medical folks, sticklers for detail, have more descriptive ways of saying things. This is from a July 2009 medical report, which gives an overview of my medical history:

> Duke is a 15-year-old male with a history of central nervous system disease associated with a cavernous hemangioma and cerebral abscess. This young boy has had multiple complications associated with a pontine cavernous angioma, which has bled twice in the past. He has been at Abbott-Northwestern Hospital from December through March of 2009 with multiple procedures, and has recently been at Gillette Children's Specialty Healthcare for rehabilitation therapy.

The report goes on and on, with many more pages of descriptive medical terminology that would almost literally drive a person's brain to bleed just attempting to read and understand it all. Try this on for size:

> He developed a diplopia, gait abnormality, and a severe headache in December, and the findings were compatible with pontine hemorrhage and hydrocephalus. He underwent a ventriculostomy and resection at Abbott-Northwestern Hospital. Surgical interventions have included resection of the pontine

cavernous angioma on 12-08-08, and on 1-02-09, he under-went gastrostomy tube placement. On 1-12-09, he underwent external ventriculostomy drainage due to hydrocephalus and pseudomeningocele. On 1-20-09, he underwent placement of a ventriculoperitoneal shunt with a Medos bowel pressure at 180 cm of water pressure. In late February, he developed wound infection of his posterior fossa incision. He had an incision and drainage of this. He grew coagulase-negative staph from the wound and has been on vancomycin. He has also been felt to have an abscess of his right cerebella hemisphere possibly due to propionibacter and has been on meropenem and vancomycin as well.

There were many positive and negative moments over the following several months. The road to medical recovery was full of momentous stops, starts, side roads, and turnarounds. A medical report of May 11, 2010, more than a year later, puts it even more in perspective. It reads in part:

Chief Complaint—Malaise and arm weakness

History of Present Illness

Mark (Duke) is a 16-year-old male with a complicated history, which started last year with a cavernous hemangioma resection and subsequent hydrocephalus and multiple complications of empyema requiring further surgery. He suffered significant neuro deficits, which include left facial droop, seventh nerve palsy, and a left eye sixth nerve bilateral gaze palsy. He also had some weakness and instability, which has required extensive physical therapy to overcome.

Recently he had an increase in his Medos valve, which he

initially tolerated well but then developed gait disturbances, pain behind the right ear, and decreased appetite. He was hospitalized last week with these symptoms and a concern for shunt malfunction. The head CT showed stable ventricles. The shunt series showed an intact shunt system. Duke improved and felt fine after hydration and Toradol.

Duke was readmitted yesterday evening (May 4) due to continued fatigue and new symptoms of shoulder weakness—unable to lift arms over his head. He retained good hand strength and dexterity. His walking was actually improved.

Past Medical and Surgical History

1. Cavernous hemangioma of the pons status post resection in 12/2008.
2. Multiple postoperative infections including wound infection, cerebellar abscess, subdural empyema, and second cerebellar abscess.
3. Status post-respiratory failure with tracheostomy and ventilator dependence—resolved.
4. Paralyzed left vocal cord.
5. Profound neuromuscular weakness more weak on the left side—improved.
6. Nystagmus of both eyes, left-eye lateral glaze palsy—6th.
7. Swallowing dysfunction—resolved.
8. Left facial droop.

I mean, why didn't someone just tell me all this, and *then* I would have known what was wrong with me? I'm just kidding of course, but you can see from the laundry list the complicated nature of my problems. It makes them impossible to describe in the shorthand, that's for sure. There were too many ins and outs, recoveries and setbacks, and crises and triumphs to enumerate here. But through it all, I survived.

I will never be able to fully express my appreciation and love for all of those who cared for me and loved me. It is also hard for me to even comprehend what had happened—and was happening—to me, or to know what I was facing ahead of me. I feel fortunate to be here today to tell my story.

To Hell and Back

Murray Eaves
Head Hockey Coach, Shattuck–St. Mary's

I MET DUKE AT A HOCKEY CAMP IN THE SUMMER OF 2006. HE WAS IN ONE of the younger groups, but a really big kid for his age, I remember. During the warm-ups, we were skating around the rink together and we started talking about him coming to Shattuck–St. Mary's.

Duke was noticed early, especially by J.P. Parise, as being a good fit for our school. Again, he was a big kid for his age, a good skater, and he could shoot the puck really well. He was a physical kid and we saw him having a great deal of potential. He was a team leader and a top player on his Bantam teams during the two years that he was with us. It is impossible to ever predict the future for a player that young, but he certainly had the potential for a bright future.

Duke had very good hockey sense on the ice. We saw excellent graduated movement in his skills from one grade to the next, and hated to see him leave to go to Hill-Murray before his freshman season.

When I heard what happened to Duke, I could really relate to it. I say that because I also had a brain stem bleed—when I was in my early forties, a little over 10 years ago. On December 12, 2001, it happened to me—the same thing. For three months, I suffered with significant issues but eventually got better. I never had to go through the surgeries and interventions that Duke has faced and gone through. Yet even now, I still have some aftereffects from the bleed, but for the most part I am doing very well. In fact, I have to mention that in many ways I feel guilty yet fortunate that I have not had to go through what has stricken Duke. My hearing and my eyes were affected, along with some other physical issues, but nothing like what Duke faced.

So, as you can see, we did have a very significant connection. We meet from time to time, and I am pretty much kept up to date as to what is going on through [Duke's father] Mark. I have seen his strength both mentally and physically. He has such a positive attitude. It is really unbelievable in so many ways. Duke is such a happy-go-lucky kid. He is always looking for a good laugh and is so personable. It is not unusual for him to go up and introduce himself to people, he is just such a nice person.

I see no difference in Duke; there is no "before" and "after." I see the same person, and I honestly don't know how he does it. I recall at his high school graduation, he was all over the place—talking to people, communicating with everyone. He was not hiding out in the back corner. He talks, laughs, living for each moment.

He has said many times that he is glad this happened to him. He speaks of there being a reason for all this to have happened, like a calling is now in place for him. I just don't see many people being able to handle it all like he has. Duke has gone through the unimaginable. He has dealt with adversity. He was on the edge of living or dying. Duke was a very popular young man when he was here at Shattuck–St. Mary's, and his popularity remains. He has not let his personal problems interfere with his living. He does not want pity. He does not want anyone to feel sorry for him.

Believe me, Duke Pieper has a story to tell and every kid should read his book, whether they have had a life-changing experience or if only to appreciate what they have and to realize how quickly it can be taken away. People may have heard what happened to Duke, but none will ever know what he has gone through. This is an opportunity for everyone to learn about life and the importance of being thankful for what we have. Even with all that was taken away from Duke, he is so very appreciative of what he has.

This is a young boy, with no better way of saying it, who has gone to hell and back. That was my description of what I went through for a few months, and he has gone through it now for more than five years. And who knows what is ahead for him?

CHAPTER 5

Who Am I?

I was living the good life, a normal teenager without a care in the world, and suddenly my life was in total disarray. I used video games to escape from the reality of what was happening and what my future held. It was a way for me to forget about my physical incapabilities.

The questions began to nag at me. *Who am I? What is going on?* My future uncertain, I looked to the lessons I had learned in the past. I have always tried to be the very best person I can be. When I was at Shattuck, we wore suits on the buses, on the planes, and in restaurants. We were respectful of others and proud of what we were accomplishing. I would say that a good part of my life I have tried to live up to that. My hockey coach at Hill-Murray, Bill Lechner, repeatedly told us, "Be respectful to others. Be a good person. Be the best you can be." Every hockey coach that I have ever had has preached that same message to me, as well as my teammates. I have heard it over and over. And I have sincerely tried to be that kind of person.

In the most dire of circumstances, I took that message to heart. I tend to ask myself, *Am I being a good person? What image am I putting out there? Am I treating others with dignity and respect?* For the most part I believe that I am trying to do the right thing. I have often been told by others that I am an inspiration because of my story, because of what happened to me and how I overcame it. I never really give that much thought, but it is nice to hear. I hope I can live up to the expectations that come with that.

When I think about being an inspiration, it intrigues me. I don't mean to pump out my chest about it, but as I look back at what I went through, I know that there are few people who have faced similar circumstances. As such, I believe that I have a responsibility to set a good example—to do the right thing and demonstrate that I have something to show others, and to help those who may have been dealt a bad card themselves. I think I can do that. I know that I want to assist others.

Sometimes I think about what happened to me and wonder who else has gone through something like this. Who has been in a hospital for nine months? Who has been paralyzed? Who has lost his ability to walk? Who has gone for two months with no clue as to what was happening to them? It's not keeping score or anything like that. What I'm saying is that I do have some credibility in this arena. I have been through the wringer and come out the other side. Helping others with their struggles is important to me and I hope I can live up to, at the very least, my own high expectations—because my expectations for myself are always high, and this is certainly no exception.

My life has taken an unusual turn, one that at times has been very difficult to accept. I would love to be playing hockey. I would love to have finished my high school years as an outstanding hockey player for Hill-Murray. I didn't even get to compete in my ninth-grade year, let alone the three other years of high school. I made the varsity and had no ice time to show for it. And football, too—one of the reasons I transferred from Shattuck to Hill-Murray in the first place. I would have loved to have had those years and those on-field accomplishments, but that ended for me, too. None of this ever happened. These are the facts, and I have had to face them head-on.

Being a good person is important to me. If I fail in that regard, I try to keep it confidential. If I think back on it and see that I was wrong, I am hurt by my own behavior. I know the difference between right and wrong, and I do my best to try to live by those standards. All around me, I have seen good people helping others by doing the right thing; they have become an inspiration for me.

It's not just helping people through tragedy. It can be the little things—like opening doors for people. I try to be nice to everyone, young and old, rich and poor, black and white and purple. Being nice to people is one of the easiest things in life to do. I think it is much harder to be rude, to be hurtful, to be unprofessional than it is to be nice. Being nice is so easy. And it's the right thing to do.

But being a good person goes far beyond opening a door or giving out a kind word; it goes much deeper. Consider this: the opportunity in school arises to cheat on a test. Depending on how the classroom is set up and what the teacher is doing, it might sometimes be quite easy to cheat. I have certainly had plenty of opportunities to cheat through the years, but I know this is wrong. How could anyone be proud of a good score on a test if they received it by cheating? It's not right, period. Things like this seem so simple to figure out, to me.

Cheating in other ways in life can often be an easy path to take. Maybe you don't record a few strokes on your golf scorecard, or maybe the cashier gives you back too much change and you keep your mouth shut. These things are so easy to do and yet so wrong. These kinds of transgressions seem so small that many people don't give them much thought, but they really define who you are and what your character is.

Life is full of little opportunities to do the right thing. I always try. I'm not always successful, but I always give it my best shot. Even with all of the medical issues that I have had and that will always be part of my life, I never let that be an excuse. They have never stood in the way of me always giving my very best in doing the right thing.

Sure, I could take a look at what happened and constantly say, "Why did this have to happen to me? What did I do to have life kick me in the face?" But that is the easy way out: Feel sorry for myself. Get sympathy from others so I can feel better. I don't do it because it doesn't make me feel better. Instead, I give it my best every single day to stay positive. Everybody has their struggles. I look at the little things in life and I'm thankful. I feel fortunate that I am where I am. It could be a lot worse.

One of the biggest steps in my life, about which I will go into more detail later, was making the decision to leave home and go off to college, at Bowling Green University in Ohio. I would be attending college in a place where I had never been before, a place where I knew no one. Some people thought it was too much. I'm sure some people wondered how realistic that much independence would be for me. As I look back, I know I made the right decision. I knew then that if I was going to get back to any form of normalcy ever again, I would have to do it on my own. I'm proud of how it has worked out. I really am. On top of everything that had happened to me, I know it did seem a little crazy. I recognize that, but for me it simply became a case of mind over matter.

My parents have done a tremendous job of encouraging me to look forward to the positive things in life. I was taught to look ahead at what is coming along next in life. What is out there? Where is the next challenge? When you hit a roadblock, what are you going to do about it? Look forward to a little vacation. Look forward to tomorrow—a game, a movie, a television show, whatever it might be. Just look ahead. Looking ahead keeps the past and the present in perspective—a positive perspective. Sometimes I have to work at it, but it is a gift to think in those terms.

I try to find things that really pump me up, and I find that it makes every day more exciting. Maybe it is an event that I am going to attend. Maybe it's tomorrow or a week away, but something out there that I know that I am going to enjoy. It's one of the things that keeps me going: thinking positively along the way.

Now, it won't be playing hockey. I know that is over for me, sad as it is. So I have to take a different approach. But maybe it's going to a game, watching other people play a sport that I truly love. That is an inspiration for me in and of itself. That's my attitude, and it works for me. As far as I see it, I don't have any other choice but to think positively—and I refuse to feel sorry for myself. I won't do it. I just won't.

Mind over matter. Take control of your own destiny. Call it whatever you like; it works. I truly believe in that concept. It works for me and it can work for others. My parents instilled good habits in me when they taught me to look ahead for the positive things. But a lot of this is me, too. I know I have to do this to move forward. When I focus my attention in that direction, it works. In reality, what choices out there are good ones, the positive ones, the ones that can move you ahead? That's what I'm always looking to identify.

If you don't have a positive attitude with what life can throw at you, you can count on being pretty much screwed. Sorry, but you are. Times are going to get tough. I have the medical records to prove it. Difficult things happen to everyone; no one is excepted. Like people say, it may get a lot worse before it has a chance of getting any better. The real question is, what are you going to do about it? How do you fight peril, tragedy, and devastation?

Someone asked me once, "How do you handle the prognosis with your disabilities?" I looked at them and politely said, "Can you put that in English?" His reply was, "I guess what I mean is, tell me how the brain bleeding has affected you and your future." The question didn't just come out of the blue; we had been talking about my medical issues. I answered him honestly and frankly. I told him that obviously I was going to have to live with what life has dealt me. I will never play hockey again. I will have double vision, problems with my facial muscles, my balance, and multiple other difficulties and disabilities. It is tough to deal with those issues moment to moment, but even more difficult to accept that they may stay with me.

I may never totally recover. Getting back to "normal" may never happen; this could be my new normal. To be honest, I have come to the realization that they most likely will never go away. I'm getting better at accepting it. What choice do I have?

My double vision is a major issue for me to overcome. I have one eye that sees in one direction, and the other sees in a different direction. Basically, when I look at something, I will see two objects instead of one. My two eyes work differently. Most people's eyes work together to form a single image. Mine don't do that. If I shut one eye, I will see one object. But there are problems that come with that as well. In addition, one of my eyes puts a slant on things. So not only do I see two objects, but one of them is askew.

Still, for the most part, I can function fairly well. But there are things that are very problematic for me; depth perception is a good example. Seeing a football coming at me and trying to catch it would be really hard to do. Trying to figure out where the ball is going to be a few seconds after I first see it is difficult. This is true for baseball, basketball, hockey, volleyball...all sports. Now add my double vision into the mix. Can you imagine that? A ball is coming in my direction, and not only do I have severe depth perception preventing me from determining where the ball actually is, but I also see two balls coming at me. It's not a good feeling to have, let me tell you. It pretty much rules out sports for me—at least at this time in my life. I am always hopeful that this will improve, but I have my doubts. I won't give up on all this, though. Never! I try to get by and do the best I can. I have someone throw three footballs to me, I might catch one. In baseball that would be pretty good in hitting, one for three.

It sounds odd, but I have conquered this issue with my driving. I have passed all the tests to drive safely because I know how to compensate. I look carefully at the cars and people around me. I overdo *everything*. I keep a close eye on the taillights of the cars in front of me to see if they are braking or not braking, that kind of thing. I have learned how to adjust, and for the most part I do very well. I try to adapt. Overall I try to cope so that I can do what every other person does in life, even if it is in a little different way. I will not let my disabilities control my life. I will fight them and conquer them. I will, and in many respects I already have. It makes me proud.

I have a new word that is paramount in my vocabulary: *adapt*. I can make things work by accepting what I am, what I have become, what abilities I have lost, and what remain. Adapt; it works.

It doesn't matter what I do from now on. I can drive. I can go to work. I can have some fun now and then with a football. The fact of the matter remains that I will have to adapt. All the things that came so naturally for me before now are not. So if I want to do those same things I did in the past, or at least some of them, I have to adapt. I have accepted this. The drive and passion I had in the past to be a great player and person helps me now in adapting to my circumstances.

Everything I do in my daily life, I do in a different way. It does not come easily. It does not come naturally. But I can do them. I will do them. I will be able to do things like everyone else, but not in the same way. I have to accept the fact that I am different now. Walking, driving, cutting the grass, picking something up off the floor or the ground...I can do it, but it takes more effort. Regardless, I will make it happen.

My vision is the chief cause of most of the problems. I have been told that if it had been muscles that were damaged, they could be restored; the optic nerve, on the other hand, doesn't work like that. I have to accept this.

In the beginning, there was a lot of feeling sorry for myself, but I have always been the type of person who would never get discouraged by a problem, no matter what it was. And what I have now is a vast problem, but I tackle it the same way. I will never give in. I will compensate. I will adapt and I will get it done. The nerves in my eyes are damaged. So what am I going to do about it?

It is what it is, and I will move on. Yet I will always keep hope alive. How could I not? In medicine, there is so much research being done on just about everything—stem cell research, research on the restoration of nerve damage. Because of this I have and will always have hope that my condition can be treated. And in the meantime, I will find my own ways to get things done and in the process try hard not to feel sorry for myself. I work at that every single day of my life. I don't know what the future holds. There is always a chance that the technology will be there for me someday. Who knows? I can look forward to something changing in my lifetime, but for now, I have had to move on, move forward, move ahead.

I am a strong person and I have a good attitude in the life I'm living right now. Before all this happened to me, I don't think I would have called myself a cocky person, but I did have a tremendous amount of confidence. I held myself to what I call a higher standard than everyone else. I don't want this to sound negative, because I don't mean it that way. I expected a lot of myself, more than most people do—at least I think I did.

I felt like I had it all going for me. I had the hockey skills, reasonably good looks, a lot of girlfriends...most everything I could have wanted at that time in my life, and I liked it. Please don't get me wrong on this. I wasn't off in my own world of glory, acting like a snob and doing foolish things. Even then I was all about doing the right thing in life, but this higher standard that I set for myself was because I had it all and I wanted to keep it and reap the rewards from it. It was not a plateau that kept me from understanding what was important in life: doing the right thing, being kind to people, and appreciating what I had. Yet I had no idea that it was all going to be taken away from me. It took so little to lose so much.

After my surgery was over and I was coherent again, I sat in my hospital bed at Abbott Hospital in Minneapolis. There was a big window in my room and I could look out and see the city, the neighborhood unfolding around us. I can recall sitting there in my wheelchair and saying to myself, "Am I ever going to be able to get back out there again? Am I ever going to be able to do what I did before, or is this pretty much it for me? Am I going to be here in this chair, like this, for the rest of my life?" Those were the kinds of things that went through my mind at the time. I didn't have any idea that things could get even worse.

What a change. There I was, this kid with everything going for me. I was this kid with the attitude that I was above everyone else in the standards that I set for myself. I had everything imaginable going for me, and then this…. There I sat in a wheelchair, looking out a hospital window and wondering, *Is this it for me?*

Sitting there in the hospital, I was not thinking I was at a standard higher than everyone else. Everything had become focused around my health. But at the same time my thinking was that I was going to get better and that I would be able to play hockey again. Deep in my mind, I was convinced this was temporary, and that hockey was still going to be part of my life again. I truly believed I would be able to be back on my team and playing again. I was wrong. Boy, was I ever wrong.

It wasn't just me. My doctor always put it in my mind that I could play hockey again. I can't recall his words exactly, but I do remember him saying something along the lines of, "Oh yeah, after the surgery, you will be able to play again." I remember those words. I held on to those words. I never really figured out the motivation behind that promise, though, because that didn't happen. Obviously.

I kept that image in my mind, of me taking the ice again. As time went on, though no one ever said it directly to me, I did face the facts. And the facts were, I was not going to play hockey again. More than that, my whole life was never going to be the same again. To say it was hard would be an understatement. Even so, it was reality.

There are times in a person's life when reality smacks you right

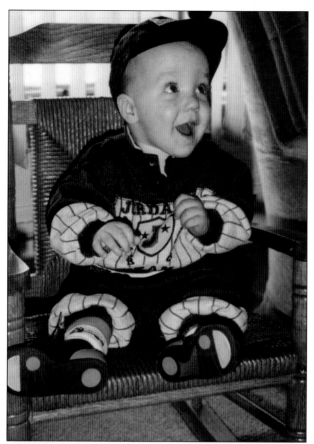

A rare sight: sitting still long enough to get my photo taken.

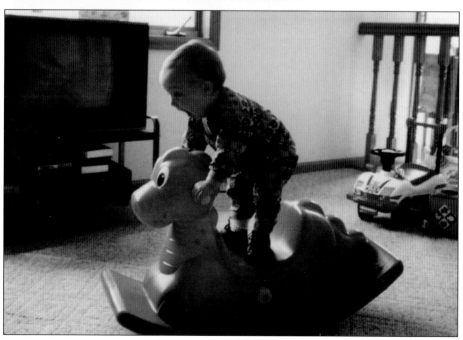

Typical daredevil stuff.

Driving heavy machinery with Dad.

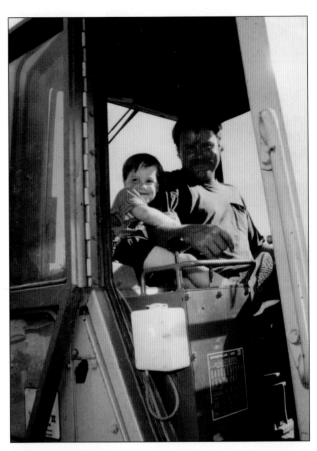

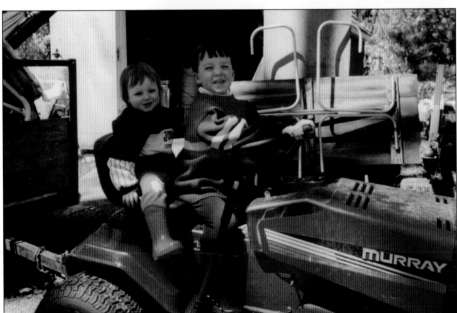

And my sister, Jackie.

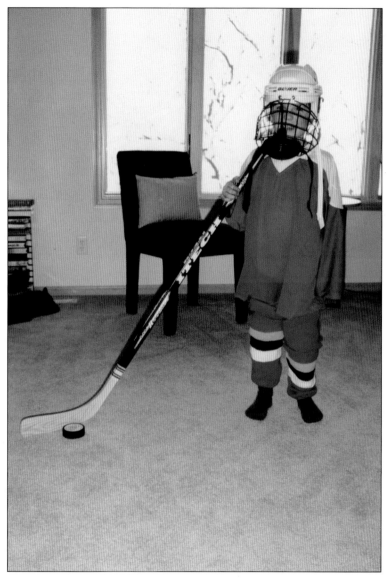

In those early days playing hockey, I just didn't enjoy putting on all that gear—or taking it off, for that matter.

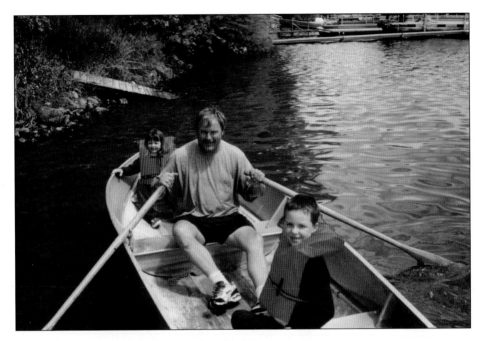

Boating at the cabin with my dad and Jackie.

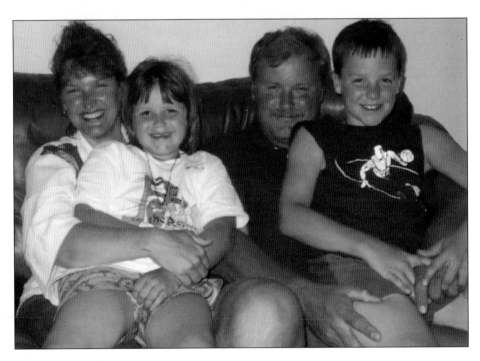

The whole family in my early years.

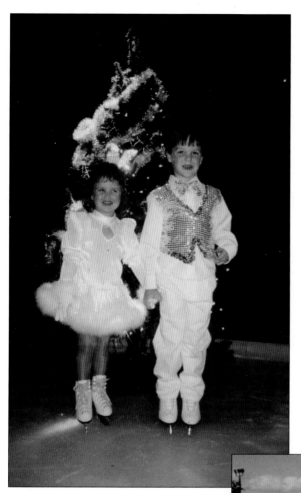

Doing ice shows was my secret hockey weapon. I was practically born on skates.

I've loved golfing since I was big enough to swing a club.

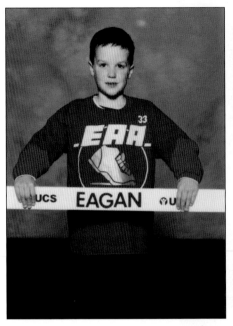
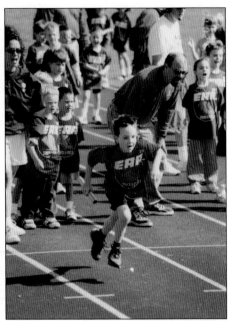

There was also track-and-field...

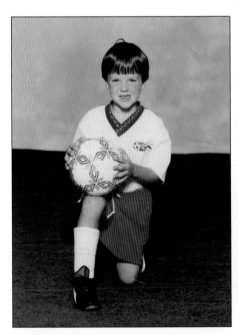
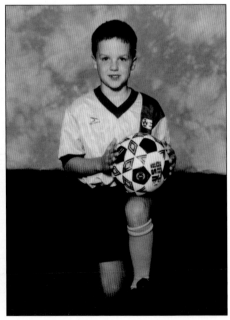

...and soccer...

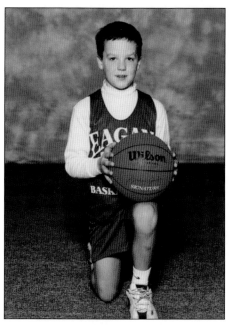

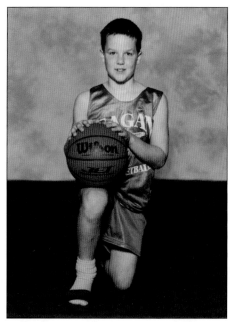

...and basketball...

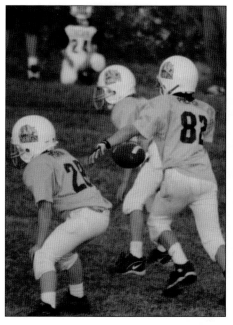

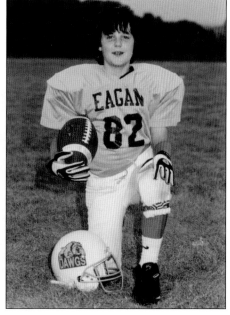

...and football.

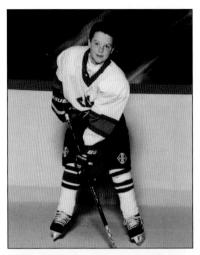
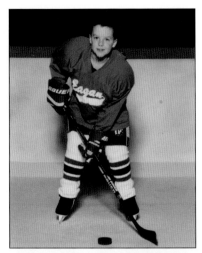
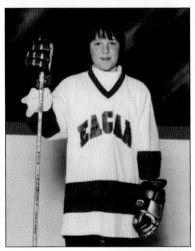
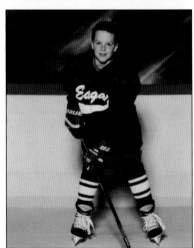
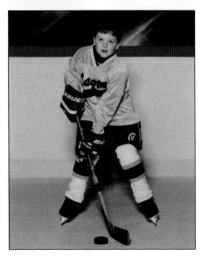

Just a few of my hockey portraits, ranging from Mini Mites to Bantams.

in the face. I had to look myself in the mirror and say, "Look, you are not going to play hockey again." I had to accept what was going on in my life. I refuse to be stupid about things. I had to face reality head-on, and I did. Dwelling on what I couldn't do wouldn't get me anywhere.

I have seen others who have not faced the realities of their own situation. When I see this, I feel sorry for them. Although there is always the possibility of a miracle recovery—and indeed, there is always a chance—the likelihood of that happening in most devastating medical occurrences is very slim. I think everyone has to be honest with themselves.

I was asked once if I think that my case is a miracle. Well, I don't know for sure, and it is hard for me to say this without sounding arrogant, but I do believe that *I* am a miracle. Now you wouldn't hear me say this in some kind of public forum or anything like that, but I do believe for me to be where I am today is a miracle. Am I in great condition now with no problems? Hardly. But to be where I am now from where I came from, yes, I do think it is miraculous. I have no question about that thought. Was there a lot of courage, a lot of hope, and a miracle, as this book title describes? I think there was, and I am eternally grateful.

It is my hope that I can use what happened to me to help others through their own difficulties. I have always been a believer in the concept that everything happens for a reason. Even after everything that happened to me, I do think that is the case. I believe that I have a calling to assist others through their medical difficulties, and I plan to do that. I am inspired by the thought. Maybe *this* is my miracle. Time will tell.

I know this. No matter what, I will do the best I can. I will give speeches about what happened to me and how I have fought through it. I will talk to others, guide them, and give my best every day. It is my goal, but it has not always been an easy mission for me. Yet I know I can do this by keeping the right attitude. I have a medical problem that will stay with me for the rest of my life. I know this. But I will never give up the fight to get what I want in life.

Some people see me, and all they see are my disabilities. When I am looked at from that kind of perspective, it's a real shame. I'm still Duke Pieper. My heart and my soul are the same, and it's too bad that part of me is now overlooked by some people. But that's their problem, not mine. I absolutely love to prove people wrong about what I can do. It is a challenge, a fight that I always intend to win. Walking, going to school, driving...everyday things that others thought I may never do again in my life. I have proved them wrong time and again and loved doing it. I will never give up. I won't stop. I love life.

I'm not sure there are a lot of people out there who knew even the basics of my situation, who would ever think that I could do what I have been able to do over the last few years. Drive with double vision? Are you kidding me? Well, I'm doing it and doing it safely. My vision today is far from normal, but I survive. You won't find me sitting in a corner and pouting about it. Not me. I will not let myself fall into that trap.

I am happy. I really and truly am. From the outside looking in, someone might take a look at me and see all my issues and problems and say, "Are you kidding me?" But I would look them right in the eye and tell them the same thing. Yes, I am happy—I have to be. There is no choice. I have to recognize and realize what my capabilities are, and determine what I can do and then make the very best of them. The realization part is important because once you accept the cards that you have been dealt, you can move on. I have, and that's a big reason why I am happy. Hope is something that is always on the table, but it needs to stay in the background; the reality of the here and now is what must be at the forefront.

I want to be a happy person and enjoy life. Hope is certainly a part of it. I love hockey and I will be linked with the game, but I know in my heart I will never play again. That is reality, and I have accepted that. But having said that, it doesn't mean I can't still be involved with the sport in other ways. I can still read about the game. I can have a few posters on the wall and I can hang with my friends who are hockey players. I am not the type to now be jealous of those who can play, or to stay away because it makes me feel bad. That is not me and that will never be me. I will always try to find a way to make the very best of my situation, and being involved with hockey is just one of the things that makes me happy.

When I was first hospitalized, I didn't go off and hide in a corner. As far as I was concerned I was still a part of the Hill-Murray hockey team. I was going to be there for my former teammates. And I was. I had to have help, but on Senior Day, I came out on the ice and met my parents. I was there. I made it. There were no goals that night, no hits, and no shots on the net, but I was there and a part of the team and the game that I love.

When it came time to think about where I was going to go to college, we had to find a place where I could fulfill my goals and love for the game, where I could continue to be around hockey. I found that at Bowling Green. The distance to get there from the day I stepped off the ice made for quite the journey, but every step has been worth it.

I find other things besides hockey that make me happy—so many other things. I mentioned my dogs before. I had a dog— one awesome dog—who invariably made me very happy, even in my darkest moments. Pepsi even visited me in the hospital on occasion. There's no doubt that I was able to get through some tough times with his help. Later, my family got another dog from my grandma, also a Wheaten Terrier, named Sprite. And we also have Crosby, a goldendoodle who is much younger.

Dogs are wonderful companions, and have been such an unwavering source of love and affection for me. I love to be around them and really enjoy the connection between us. They have alleviated so much of my pain. They listen to me. I can tell them my troubles. At the same time, I am saying to myself, "What are you going to do about this? Do I like how I feel today or at this moment?" I guess the fact is if you have enough of the wherewithal to ask that kind of question of yourself, obviously things are not going well for you, and the answer will always be "No." "No, I don't like how I feel today." But the real question is, "So what am I going to do about it?"

Being around the people that I love is another huge source of happiness, and I can't imagine a family better than mine. I am extraordinarily grateful. And being able to do what I like to do, even the simple things, makes me happy. I think people in life have to find their niche, whether it be with family, friends, pets, or doing what you enjoy. Making the most of our opportunities makes life enjoyable and wholesome.

Sadness, unfortunately, is also a part of life. I have gotten pretty good at handling this, especially when I reflect upon what has happened to me. I'm not like other people anymore. The harsh reality is that I'm not like my friends or other kids my age, and I never will be again.

As I said before, I have accepted this, but there are still times when sadness creeps into my life. I guess it is inevitable given the circumstances of what I face every day. Sometimes it will creep in on me at night, when I am lying in the darkness. When I think about never being able to play hockey again—let's just say that especially in the beginning, I have to be honest, it was not an easy ride.

I know that it sounds simple to say that you just have to move on and accept what life has given you, but the reality is that the ride does have a lot of peaks and valleys, and I have had to fight off the sadness often. Playing hockey was my life and I loved every aspect of the game, every single part of it. And to have it taken away from me—well, it has not been easy to cope with on top of everything else.

I was a good player on top of enjoying the game. Most of my friends played hockey. I thought I would leave high school, go on to play college hockey, and someday play in the National Hockey League. That was my goal, my dream, and where I saw my life going. And it is gone.

When sadness does rear its ugly head, I fight it with everything I have. Mind over matter. That's my best defense, and it makes good sense to me. I find ways to handle it.

Girls are another matter, another arena in which I have to adapt. Before, I definitely had an active social life. Girlfriends, yeah, I always seemed to have one. I recall Jackie saying, "My brother, Duke, he always has a girlfriend." I used to laugh and enjoy hearing her say that. I had lots of dates—mostly just groups of us hanging out. We went to movies sometimes, or hung around the park near our house. They were good times, always among friends.

Since my medical problems, it has been more difficult. I don't look the same, talk the same, or act the same. I am the same person at my core. And in some ways I think I changed for the better. I think my heart is bigger. I think I accept people more for who they are and not what I think they should be. I know that I am one in a million considering what happened to me, and I look at it in a positive way. I try to think, *Who wouldn't want me? I'm special.*

The easiest thing to do in life when you are smacked in the face like I have been is to give up. Just plain throw in the towel and give up. Believe me, I have felt that way plenty of times. Plenty of times.

There are days when things aren't going your way. We all have those days—some are for good reason and others are...well, just because. For me, I suppose maybe I have had more than my fair share. Things would sometimes get worse than the day before, and then when you think things can't get any worse, they do. I recall times when I thought things were on the upturn, when I began to feel better and thought I was getting better, then *BAM*, more surgery. I kept thinking, *Are you kidding me? When is this all going to end? I don't like needles, I don't like hospitals, and I don't like signing papers for more surgery.* But there I was, doing it all over again. It was just awful.

There were also times when I really didn't know what was going on. I remember once being really angry at one of my doctors. I felt like he was just in the business of ordering people around. I guess some people call it a "poor bedside manner." I felt like he wasn't asking me a lot of questions or giving me any sympathy. In his brusque way, he'd come in and say, "Just do this. Just do that. Put your John Hancock on this document." It really ate at me.

My uncle was the one who got me through this period when he told me, "Look, Duke, at least he knows what he is doing. He isn't asking a lot of questions because he knows what needs to be done." Basically, "This guy knows what he is doing and what has to happen to help you." It helped me a lot to hear that, and it calmed me down and made me better. Tough times? There were plenty of them.

When things got worse, it was my family who got me through. Them and that whole "mind over matter" thing. I was able to find a way to get through it, to fight and survive through any means possible.

I was asked once to describe how I have changed after everything that has happened to me. My answer was simple and to the point: "Drastically." From the physical standpoint, it's quite simple. I cannot do most of the things in life that I used to do, at least not in the way I did them before. I have had to learn how to do many things basically from scratch.

Mentally and emotionally, I have learned to accept what has happened to me. Additionally, I have learned to accept more people into my life. What I mean by that is that my circle of friends and connections to others has expanded. Before, I never had a lot to do with the nonathletic type of kid—the "nerds," I suppose, is another way of putting it. It wasn't that I wasn't interested in getting to know other people, it's just that my circle of friends was so insular. Now, I have to admit I hang around all kinds of groups. Everyone seems to fit in.

Some of my old friends are still in my life, but some of my closest contacts and friends are different now than they were a few years ago when I was strictly connected to the hockey players. This, I know, is a good change for me. I have accepted people for who they are, and I am very proud of this.

Maturity often comes with age, but I think it can also come from a life-changing experience. In my case, I know it can change you for the better. You realize what the important things in life are, and in many instances they are your friends and family. A person can be a great athlete, get a lot of attention, and feel really good about what they may have accomplished on the ice or the field, but I have learned there is another important side of life. That is something I am recognizing now, and I feel lucky to know it.

Luck has entered my life along with many other things. When you look at my situation, it is easy to say, "Wow, he really got dealt a bad hand," but I don't look at it that way. I look at things from a different perspective. I feel lucky. A million things could have gone wrong. Things could have been far worse. I could have died, for one thing! But I didn't, and I sincerely believe that what happened and how I have survived is all for a reason. And for whatever reason, this was supposed to happen to me. Today I have somewhat of an idea what that reason might be, but I am confident that as I move through life, it will become even more clear. I truly do believe this. I am a strong believer in God and I have a lot of faith. Things happen for a reason. I am positive about this, and that is why I now have to accept what has happened to me and fully explore all the reasons why. I have to find out my purpose.

To be totally honest, at the time of my hospitalization, I had a crisis in my life. I always thought I had some kind of connection with God. Even to the point that, when I was going into surgery for the first time, I had faith that I was going to be fine. Well, I wasn't fine. And after my first two months in the hospital, how couldn't my faith have been shattered?

I used to talk to God regularly. I prayed. I went to Communion. I did all the right things because my faith was strong. And then look what happened. There was a time when I can honestly say that I felt, why wouldn't I hate God, hate my faith, and feel that none of it was worthwhile? I went through that stage, and I understand it now. I am past that now because I know there was a reason, and it will become a platform in my life for who I am and what I am. It will be a guidepost for what I do in my life and it will provide an even stronger faith than I had before my incident.

Getting myself straight with God was a long process. I thought many times, *Why me? Why did you do this to me? We had this great thing going between us, God, and now look what happened. Why me? I mean, what the hell?*

I got past it. I do not have these feelings anymore and have not had them for a long time. I have dealt with my crisis of faith. It wasn't easy, but I realized I had to get past those thoughts and feelings because it became so obvious to me that you will never get anywhere in life being angry at everyone, especially God. What would be the point of going on like that? It won't ever move you forward, only bury you in misery and hatred. So I buried those thoughts—the anger, the recrimination, the self-pity—and I moved on with the foundational belief that all of this happened to me for a reason. God engineered it. I manned up, accepted the challenges that lay ahead of me, and acted. So far, I think I am doing a pretty good job.

As I said, I truly believe that people who go through life-changing experiences have to not only accept the challenges ahead for themselves, but also look to the future in a positive way, as difficult as that may be. Hope will always be there too. It has to be. For me, there is always an element of hope in every part of my future. In reality, however, I know I won't be running any marathons or winning any golf matches or skating the way I once did. I know that and have accepted it. I have accepted my fate and plan to use it as a stepping stone to my future.

It is what it is. I am what I am: different from before, but with a new acceptance, a new fight, and a positive outlook on what is to come.

CHAPTER 6

I Just Can't Cry Anymore

I have cried so much that it feels like I cannot shed another tear. I don't think there is anything left in me. Sometimes it was out of discouragement, or a sense of loss, or frustration. I mean, look what I had and lost. I'm not sure this is easy for anyone to understand unless one has personally gone through it. Yes, sure, I did have a tough time. And there was a time when I didn't handle it very well. I had my moments, sure. Who wouldn't? Most of the time I was mad at God and my parents. *Mad*, I suppose is not an adequate word to describe how I actually felt. In some ways, I was just plain angry with the whole world. And I felt like I had to find *someone* to blame for all my troubles.

I have cried so many times over my injury/episode—I have a lot of different names for it—that I couldn't even begin to count. I have cried because I can't do what every other person can do, something I used to be able to do and maybe took for granted. I have cried because of my new appearance, my inabilities, what I have missed in my past, my future, and a million other things. Yet crying is no longer an option for me.

I have come to the conclusion that crying is a waste of time. The facts are facts, and no amount of self-pity will change them. If I spend all my energy feeling sorry for myself, it won't make me see better, walk better, or play hockey again. Instead, that energy could be put to another, more productive use.

Not too long ago, I caught a show on television about hockey championships. At one point, it showed a team win the Stanley Cup championship in the NHL. One of the players on the ice was skating around, holding the Stanley Cup over his head in celebration. This was my dream, playing out right before my eyes. This is what I was going to do someday. As I was watching it, that very thing echoed in my head. *This is what I am supposed to be doing someday. This is my dream.* And then, reality: *And now it is all gone.* At one time, when crying was a viable option for me, something like this would have broken me down, made me blubber like a child and feel sorry for myself. But what would be the use? It wouldn't change a thing, not one bit.

When these kinds of experiences blindside you—and they will—you have to find a way to get through those moments. You have to find a way within yourself to let it pass. When that TV show ended, I can recall turning off the television and immediately putting my mind to something else. It does absolutely no good to dwell on something that you have no power or ability to change. So if you cannot do anything about something, no matter how big or small, then forget it. Move on.

I think you learn over time how to handle sadness and despair. The more it enters your life, the better you get at coping with it. There are all kinds of reminders out there every single day for me:

things I used to be able to do and will never be able to do again. I have to find ways to get past those moments, and I usually can. It makes everything much easier.

I know from experience that the right strategies for handling every one of these kinds of issues will not always come right away. It takes a while to learn to deal with reality. As time has gone by, I have become better at it. I have had more practice. These days, I get over things easily. And crying is not an option; I have taken that off the table for myself.

My mom and dad have helped me a lot through these tough times. I have seen how much they care about me, and their virtues have rubbed off on me. I have seen what they have sacrificed for me. I appreciate it more than they can ever imagine. Their generosity and their love gives me no choice but to show them and myself that I can move ahead and live a positive and productive life. The profound love that they have shown me, and continue to show, is incredible. I would not have made my way out of the sadness and despair without their help.

The drive that my dad has had, working 24/7 and still being there for me when I need him, has been so inspirational to me. Dad works all the time. He has shown me about setting goals and refusing to quit. I got that drive from him. His loyalty, love, commitment, and caring are the attributes I hope I can mirror when I have my children.

I was 15 years old when everything happened to me. A few years have gone by, and in many ways I have been through a lot. But I am still young—just a kid, really—and I have a great deal to look forward to in my future. I am just beginning to live my life. I have so much ahead, and I will not let anything get in the way, least of all my own attitude. Sure, I have been knocked down some. I will never be a Stanley Cup champion. I will never play college hockey, let alone professionally. So what?

I have learned a lot in the past few years. I have grown up. I can see the bigger picture. There is a lot more to life than hockey. At one point in my life, I'll admit that I was not sure there was anything more important, but what happened to me has been an eye-opening experience. There is so much more, and I am going to explore it. There is a whole new world out there for me to find and enjoy.

There have been other things that have motivated me besides my family. I have always looked forward to going to college. And although I thought my college years would be all about playing hockey, I know now that there is so much more to higher education than that. Experiencing college life was something I did not want to miss out on. It became a motivation for me to get there. Certainly I was not going to dwell on whatever restrictions in life might keep me from doing it.

But let's get even more elemental. Take walking, for example. It is such a given in life for most people. You don't even give it a thought, just get up in the morning and go. It's so simple. Most people only have a first time learning how to walk, when they are very young. Some lose the ability to do it when they are very old. But I was neither young nor a baby. I lost the ability to walk as a teenager, and I was forced to learn it all over again. Previously I could skate around an ice rink almost as if I were on air. I had speed, I had agility, I had coordination. I had all the tools I needed to be successful. And then I didn't have any of that. But I learned that skill, like so many other things, all over again.

Finishing high school, my college life ahead—those things motivated me. I had a drive to get out of that wheelchair and walk. I hated the position that I was in, and it had to change. I was going to walk. I refused to live the rest of my life looking out a window from a wheelchair. And as difficult as it was, I did it. I learned how to walk again, one step at a time.

In the midst of the serious medical struggles I was going through, a funny thing happened to me. I started to really pay attention to what others around me did, and took time to really listen to and watch others. One thing I noticed is that a lot of people are really negative. They find the time in their day to complain about things. These are people who have their health, who have their bodies, who do most anything they want to do. I became really annoyed hearing their complaints about the little things, things that are meaningless in the grand scheme of life—at least from my perspective and in comparison to what I was facing. It just seems to me that a lot people are so much quicker to complain about the things going wrong in their lives than to be thankful for the good things. Why is that?

Play golf? Play baseball? Play football? Play hockey? Skate? Run? No, I don't think so, not for me. It's over for me. Yet you complain because it's raining outside. The weather is too cold. Your stick isn't taped properly. Your blades are dull. The ice is soft. Are you kidding me? These are things that I would hear from people from time to time that would drive me crazy! But I never really let it get to me or occupy much of my time. Suffice it to say, it really put life in perspective. It taught me how much in life we take for granted, something that often doesn't sink in until it is taken away.

Once in a while a scenario would pop into my head that would kind of get me irritated and put into perspective the contrast between how I now look at things compared to some others. For example, let's say that someone is headed for work in the morning and on the way to an important meeting. They get stuck in traffic, then get a flat tire, end up being late for work, and miss the meeting. The entire morning is a mess for them: gridlock, a flat tire, late arrival, a blown meeting—more than a tripleheader of a bad day, right?

Well, compared to me not being able to physically move (or do anything) for two months...well, see what I mean? You think you are having a bad day? Take a look at me.

It is a good lesson, no question about that. However, I have figured out that it does no good for me to get upset and dwell on what others do. It serves no purpose for me. For others, it might, but I doubt it. I think that if they would get their heads out of their behinds, they would be a lot happier and realize what the important things in life are. "So you think you are having a bad day? Well, you have nothing to speak of compared to what I have going in my day," I'd tell them. "You can move, talk, eat, sleep. You can do whatever you want. I can't move. I can't breathe on my own. I can't do anything that you can do. And you're having a bad day? I don't think so."

There are frustrations that I experience every day. I know this and understand it and even expect it. There is no doubt that with all the difficulties that I face each day, the biggest thing for me is no longer being able to play sports. Sports were basically my life when this all happened to me. I tried to do a few things after the fact. When I was in a wheelchair, I could throw the ball around a little; I could play a little wheelchair basketball. It wasn't the same, but it helped. I suppose that if I practiced a lot I could probably throw a ball close to the way I used to do it. Catch a ball, probably not. Considering my double vision, that would be much more of a challenge. Double vision in itself causes so many difficulties on a constant basis. It affects every single thing I do. When it comes to sports, it makes things almost impossible.

I remember early on at college, there was a midnight skate event, which was followed by a massive broom ball game. The old Duke would have jumped at the chance, but unfortunately both were out for me. I couldn't do it. In the past, it would have been a great time. I would have enjoyed every second of it.

Still, I have made great improvements since the beginning of my recovery. I have improved my motor skills by leaps and bounds. And I have greatly improved my attitude and learned to accept my status. I hope to someday be able to participate to some extent in skating, football, and some of the other things I mentioned earlier. If I work at it and practice certain things hard enough, I can eventually learn how to do them again. It's tough, but I'm really motivated to get my life back.

I've already had so much success getting my skills back. Take walking, for example; that came back. Eating, ditto. Breathing came back. Drinking, that too. My double vision remains, but I have been able to work around it. So, many of my basic skills have returned, and I am very thankful and appreciative to be where I am today. Considering where I came from, unable to do anything, I have come a long way. None of it comes without a great amount of effort and determination. I just listed a very few things that most people do by routine and that for me are a struggle. Make no mistake, I could list a million more things that most people take for granted every day and that I will never again. A million more.

My coordination continues to be a problem, but I am working on it. My balance is okay most of the time, but I still have a lot of work to do. It is—I am—a work in progress. I understand this, and it is a very important thing for me to acknowledge. Every single day is a new opportunity for me to improve my skills, and I will never give in to grief and despair. I know I have the ability to improve on things a little bit every single day, and I remain committed to doing that.

I keep a positive attitude. Believe me, I know it is not possible to get through those things in life that smack you in the face without occasionally getting discouraged. No one can do that. I try to keep a positive attitude as much as I can. Sometimes it is tough, but it is a huge goal of mine.

I would never have improved to the point where I am today without a positive outlook; I know that. I know that I didn't do it alone. I had tremendous assistance from my family, from God intervening, among other things. I think there probably are some people that have gone through difficulties like I have who have left that despair. You have to leave it. Mind over matter helped me, but the point is that you have to keep searching until *something* works. Staying in a negative zone is one of the most dangerous places you can be.

My parents really were there for me to give me the boost I so sorely needed. My mom was there for me for just about everything. She was a 24/7 mom and basically handled every one of my needs for me. My dad provided spiritual inspiration and emotional support. The two of them were so instrumental to me during that time, and they remain special to me. They were there, helping me through the toughest times.

When all this happened to me, I was basically isolated from the rest of the world. I was at home, doing homeschooling for a period of time, so I never saw my friends in school. I was also inundated with physical therapy, both at the hospital and later at home. It was almost too much to take on, but I got through it.

At the hospital, I would have quite the day trying to do the things that had once come so naturally to me. I was starting over from square one. While my friends were at school and playing the sports that I loved and laughing with friends and chasing girls, I was toiling to learn the basics in life all over again.

My typical day began with a physical therapy walking session in the morning. As I walked, my mind wandered to the used-to-be. I had made the Hill-Murray varsity hockey team as a freshman. It was going to be the beginning of a fabulous high school hockey career: four years at a great school and then off to college. And football, that was going to be a big part of it, too. Then the hockey pros after that, if I got good enough. I already had some colleges that had taken an interest in me. I would reflect on those things, wander off into my dream world. *Places like Bowling Green were interested in me coming there to play hockey.* And then, *STOP! STOP! STOP!* Not going to happen. I mean, I was in the hospital taking walking lessons in the morning as part of my day. *Walking lessons!* College scholarships…the NHL…that was gone.

After my walking lessons, I would have a short break and then it was on to occupational therapy. There I learned how to comb my hair, brush my teeth, and do many of the basic skills that I had lost the ability to perform.

I dreaded the walking session. I *hated* it. Even to this day, I can't understand how others can do it so easily. I know that I will never actually be able to explain this to the level that I want to explain it, but I will give it a try. I look at how easily people do things like walk, stand, move—all the simple things. I can't understand how they could do these things with such ease. I constantly used to ask myself why I couldn't do those things myself. I mean, I would look at people who were out of shape. I would look at people who were old. I would look at people with no muscle mass and think to myself, *Why is this so difficult for me to do? Look at them. They don't even think about what they are doing. I mean what in the hell is going on here? Here I am in great shape physically, a conditioned athlete, someone who has always taken care of his body, and look at me. I can barely do anything!* It was so frustrating.

The challenge in doing things like walking, standing, and sitting wasn't that it hurt. It wasn't painful to do. I just couldn't do it. I had no balance. It felt like my muscles had deserted me. My innate athletic abilities had left me completely. I don't know where they went, but they sure weren't where they used to be. Looking at others doing the simple things, I would sometimes be bitter: *Why can that person do what I used to be able to do when I can't anymore? It's not fair!* I now know how people feel when they are in a wheelchair. It hurt me so much that I could not do what I used to be able to do.

But through all the struggles I endured—and still endure on a daily basis—there is one thing as important as anything else, and that is that I am extremely thankful that I survived. I have so many opportunities for achievement in my life. I have come a long way after my brain injury, and I am very grateful to have the opportunity to continually improve my condition and abilities. My mental condition has improved along with my physical condition. As far as I'm concerned, they go hand in hand; one is connected to the other.

Enduring those very tough times wore me out physically and mentally. And those really tough times brought about a lot of tears, but I have moved on. I don't think there are any tears left. So I can't cry anymore.

"We Want You with Us"

Bill Lechner
Head Hockey Coach, Hill-Murray High School

I FIRST MET DUKE PIEPER THROUGH HIS UNCLE NICK GARIBAY, WHO WAS an outstanding hockey player at Hill-Murray. Nick's sister is Duke's mom. He was from Edina and Duke grew up knowing about his uncle's connection to Hill-Murray, so I'm sure that is where the interest came from in wanting to attend school here.

Duke was at Shattuck playing hockey, and during the summer prior to his ninth-grade year. I received a phone call from Nick, who informed me that his nephew was interested in attending Hill-Murray and wanted to come out and look around. That was the first time I knew about Duke. I learned at that time that he had been at Shattuck, because it is not our way to go around snooping to recruit kids for our school; I just don't do that. Nick was a friend, so when he called, I welcomed their visit.

My first thought was, *Why would Duke want to come here when he lives in Edina where they have a great hockey program?* I also wondered why he would want to leave Shattuck. But having said that, I also thought, *If he wants to come here, we would love to have him.*

I brought him around the school. We talked about sports and I learned about his background and a little more about his family. I knew his mom somewhat, as she was a figure skating instructor and my daughter was involved in figure skating, so there was another connection there.

Duke liked Hill-Murray enough on our brief visit to enroll in the fall of his freshman year. I thought from the beginning that he was a very nice young man, very polite with very good manners. He was the type of kid who would shake your hand, look you straight in the eye, and have good conversation with you. That's the way he was built: very mature for an eighth-grader coming in as a freshman.

Physically I saw a young man who was more mature than the average kid who comes here at that young age. So I saw a good kid, a polite kid, and someone who looked to be a good athlete. And on top of that, his uncle Nick, whom I knew and trusted, told me, "Bill, Duke is real. He is a good kid."

Duke played football that fall and I got to know him better as the school's athletic director. I would see him around the school, in the halls, and talked with him from time to time. When hockey season came around, we had our regular tryout week. My philosophy has been to give the freshmen a chance to make the varsity if they prove to be good enough. I do not give special favors to anyone because of whom they know or whom I know. If they are good enough, they will have a shot at making the team, even though it is highly unusual for a ninth-grader to make the varsity.

I was with the kids for tryout week. There had been captains' practices without the coaches, but we basically had one week of tryouts to determine our team for that year. We generally have about 80 to 90 kids trying out for the varsity, with only 20 making the roster. That year was even more of a challenge to make the varsity because we had been state high school champions in the previous season and had most of the team returning. So to crack the varsity lineup that particular year was even more difficult.

We keep an open mind, and everyone has a legitimate chance to make it. In Duke's case, even though he had Uncle Nick, it did not mean anything as far as whether he was going to be selected. We keep friends and relatives and we cut friends and relatives. That is the way we are built and the way we do things here. If they have talent, we want them. We want to win.

When my assistant coach, Pat Schafhauser, and I looked at Duke, our initial thoughts were, *He is a pretty good player for a young kid.* We have had a lot of experience with this and know that if we see a young player who cannot handle the size, speed, and competition of the older kids, we get them out of that environment rather quickly. We know that a young kid can get hurt easily and we are very careful to protect our players and put them among those of their abilities.

In Duke's case, with all the initial drills, he did great. He held his own very well with the older, more seasoned players. On Wednesday of tryout week, he did very well in the scrimmage and we thought, *This kid can play.* And by Thursday we knew that we had to keep him on the varsity. He was that good.

Duke had the physical skill to handle it. He had the physical frame and the skills to make the team. No question, he was raw, a young talent, but he was a player. He was one of the top six defensemen that we kept.

Pat was a former professional player who was injured and paralyzed after being hit from behind during a game. His responsibility was to work with the defense, so he worked closely with Duke. Later, he had a connection with Duke because of their similar medical situations. Pat coaches from a wheelchair. He has been with me for more than 15 years. The two of them had a great connection.

We have a tradition at the school that happens right after tryouts, which is that we immediately take the team for some practice scrimmages on the road. This kind of alleviates some of the pressure and tension for those who made the team and also those who did not. It is a very tough time for all involved, and we have always felt that getting away for a few days helps to simmer things somewhat. There are a lot of emotions going around, from excitement to disappointment. I mean, 40-some kids did not make the varsity, and a good number of others did not make the junior varsity either.

We get on a bus the following morning and head up north to scrimmage some of the northern schools, like Grand Rapids, Hibbing, and all the other teams that we can. This gives the players a chance to get to know each other and do a little team bonding. Duke was with us. He was very much accepted by the older kids. He had a good personality and fit in extremely well. I observed this, and it was good to see how well he was received by the older players.

We were about a week before the first game of the season and had been involved in three separate scrimmages. We took a good look at Duke and he did well. With a young player such as Duke, we were watching to see if he could handle the physical part of the game. Could he hold his own out there, or would we have to come back and send him to the junior varsity? He held his own. Duke did well.

We had a very skilled hockey team at the time, and all we expected of Duke was that he do his job and let the seasoned players do theirs. And he handled this very well. He did a good job.

As far as where he stood with the defense, usually four or five of the six defensemen play on a regular basis. Duke was by no means at the bottom rung; he was going to play. We saw early on that this kid was good enough that he was going to get some pretty regular playing time. We thought, based on his abilities and time, that the sky was the limit for him. We felt that we were going to get four good hockey years out of him and then, with his high school diploma, he would go on to play for a Division I school, which was one of his goals.

So we had the week of practices and scrimmages and were ready for our first game. Now I need to say something here, and it is not arrogance and I am not trying to be corny or anything like that. But I do think in some sort of religious way that God or someone helped me to realize that Duke was in trouble before the first game. In the old days, it seemed like we would usually handle a situation like what was to develop with Duke by simply saying, "Look, get some water. You'll be fine. It's okay." (There just were not the precautions that we have today.) But not this time.

I can remember the moment as if it was this morning. We had just been state champions and we were playing Burnsville, so the game was being televised by Fox Sports North. There was a lot building up to the opening game.

Duke was out there, playing his first varsity game. He had his Hill-Murray jersey on and it was a big deal, it really was. After warm-ups, I recall he came in, but to that point had not said that anything was wrong. I later learned that during the day he had been having some vision and balance issues, but to the point when he came up to me in the locker room, I knew nothing about his physical problems.

I'm sure he was trying to fight through it, thinking it was nerves or whatever. I mean, he is just a kid. Right after warm-ups he came up to me, and I can picture the exact spot where he was standing, and he said, "Coach, I'm dizzy. There is something wrong. I can't seem to focus." Again, my first impression was, *Well, you're a freshman. You're scared to death. You are just a puppy. The game is on television,* all that. My brain was saying, *You're fine. Take some water and go.* But there was something in my brain that was telling me, *No, this is weird. We better err on the side of caution.* Normally, at home, we have a trainer with us who has been around 15 to 16 years and who I could trust to take a look at him and assess what the problem was. But on this night, we were on the road and he wasn't with us.

I didn't know the Burnsville trainer, but we still had Duke looked at, and we really couldn't figure out what the problem was at that point. There is always the pressure to win, and the easy thing to do would have been to just say, "Okay, be hurt tomorrow, but we need you tonight. So let's go and play." But as I said, there was something inside telling me that was not the way to go. I told myself, *You know what? We need to find out about this and see what is wrong.*

Duke really wanted to play, I could tell, but we needed to be cautious. At that moment, our thinking was to shut things down, thinking at the time that he would have plenty of games to play in the future and that he would have a long career ahead of him. Obviously we didn't know the serious condition that he was in that night.

Duke took off his skates and went to find his dad. Keep in mind, while this was all going on we were still committed to play the game. The ice was being surfaced. I had to talk to the team and do other things, so things were somewhat chaotic before the game.

We had little idea at the time that his situation was as serious as it turned out to be. I honestly believed that he would have whatever the problem was taken care of and that he would be back with us, probably the next day, and by the next game for sure. Of course, I later found out that would not be the case. In fact, when we learned how serious his situation was with his brain stem, it was a frightening thought to think that he might have played in the game and gotten hurt. It was a rough game and he likely would have been knocked around, and in the condition he was in, I shudder to think what the results could have been.

Once I learned what his condition was, I was so thankful that he did not play, that the something telling me *This is more serious than it looks* was real. In my younger coaching days at maybe 24 or 25 years old, I may have been the coach saying, "You're okay. It will be fine.

Now let's go out there and win this thing." I might have been that guy. I am so thankful I was not that night.

I think that as you get older and have a family, have your own kids, you get smarter. You balance the things in life that take precedence over other things. We learn as we age and get more experience. There are two ways to go with these situations. One way is to say, "Hey, toughen up, kid." Obviously the better way is, "Hey, let's be smart about this and take the cautious route."

Later, according to various sources, we were told that if Duke had played and been hit in the right place, the results could have been fatal. I mean, this was Hill-Murray versus Burnsville—high school hockey at its best. It was going to be a rough-and-tumble game, no doubt. And it was.

Mark Pieper called me the next day and told me what was happening with Duke. All I could think was, *Oh, no.* And then it became a roller-coaster ride for Duke. One day we would hear one thing and then the next day something else. "He is going to make it." "He is not going to make it." "He is going to make it." "He is going to be paralyzed." I mean, it was incredible, and so sad.

I had contact two to three times a week. You know, we are all competitive and we want to win and fill the trophy cases. It's what we do. But the real truth to all of this is, we love the kids. Something like this really hits home to coaches and those connected to the programs. I know it sure did with me.

Duke was only a freshman on the team, but he was such a good kid, a really likeable kid. He fit in so well with everyone. The team really didn't know how to handle it at first. It was kind of like, *Well, he broke his arm. He had a few stitches. He will be back in a few days.* I don't think most of the kids could even comprehend the serious nature of what Duke was going through and facing for the future.

As time went on, I think most of the guys began to realize how serious this all was for Duke and his family. Still, to fully understand the details was difficult. There were so many surgeries over the months that I'm not sure most of us truly understood what it all meant. Was his condition temporary, permanent, or what? I think everyone honestly felt that at some point he would be back playing for us again. I think at first we thought maybe by Christmas, then maybe by the next season. At some point, though, the reality set in as to the long-term nature of what he was going through.

At least twice I can remember crying, and feeling honored at the same time, when Duke's father called and asked me to do something for Duke. "Bill, Duke really, really has learned to love you. If he passes away, will you be a pallbearer for his funeral?" he asked me. I did not want to have these conversations. Although I felt so incredibly honored, I would tell Mark, "I don't want these conversations. He is going to get better. Duke is going to get better."

I cannot imagine what his family was going through at the time. All the emotions, the ups and downs, setback after setback. It had to be absolutely unbelievable.

I went to see him quite often with Pat, my assistant coach. It seemed like every time we went the room was filled with doctors. Duke was wired to everything, had monitors all over him, and at times there must have been five or six medical staff in the room. It was amazing. I had never seen anything like that before in all my hospital visits in the past. It was a real eye-opener. It was a scary experience. I have been around sports and injuries, serious kinds of situations, my whole life, but I can honestly say I had never seen anything quite like that.

Over the years, Duke and I have had contact—not as much as I would like, but time does go on. It makes me feel guilty that I don't see

Duke as much as I would like, but he is away at school. I understand; he understands.

After the incident, he was going to be homeschooled for about two years and then he wanted to come back to Hill-Murray for his junior and senior years. It took a combined effort by Hill-Murray and the Edina school system so that things would all mesh together for his return, so that he could graduate on time with his class. It was a challenge, and I give a real hats off to both systems for making it all work out. It was kind of ironic because the two schools, Edina and Hill-Murray, are always competing for hockey supremacy, but on this one, the schools worked hard together for Duke.

It was pretty cool when Duke came back to school. I first saw him about an hour after he was here. I knew he was coming. It was really neat. We could see some of the issues right away with him, such as his balance, but it was just great to have him back.

It was very difficult for the kids. Kids are kids. For many, they didn't know quite how to react, what to say—that kind of thing. For some of the hockey players who knew him, it was a little easier, but then they were moving on. Duke was great, as he has always been.

One of our best athletes here at the time, Zach LaValle, was a great leader through all this. He stuck with Duke through everything. He was the type of kid to be there when needed, and he sure was.

Duke was involved again with the hockey program when he returned. I told him when he was ready he could join the team and help out in any way that he could. Obviously, he was not going to play again, but we wanted him around with us. I even told him, "If you can play again, you will be with us. If you can't play, you will be a team manager. When you are a senior, you will be one of the team captains. Your senior year, we will not have two captains, we will have three, and you will be one of them. You will wear your jersey. No one else will wear it, and on Senior

Night, you will put on that jersey and go out with the team. We want you with us." I wanted him to feel a part of the team.

I was amazed right from the beginning by what he was able to accomplish. With all the problems he has, to learn that he got his driver's license was absolutely incredible. I used to kid him all the time by telling him, "Duke, I love you and that is fantastic that you got your license, but stay away from my car, would you, please? I don't even like one door ding. When you are driving, please stay away from me. Don't park near me. Stay at least one street away." "Oh, Mr. Lechner!"

Senior Night at Hill-Murray is always a special night for the kids, and it takes place before the last home game. It is a night to honor the players who have been on the hockey team and are seniors, playing in their last regular-season home game. It is a really special night for the players and for their families and friends. It has been a longtime tradition.

Duke had to be helped onto the ice by two of his teammates. It was sad to see. You can never say anything is guaranteed, but Duke had the potential to be a big-time hockey player. There are always players who hit a plateau, but I really feel that he would have definitely played Division I college hockey and likely would have had the opportunity to show his skills later on. He was a big, strong, tough kid.

I have been so wonderfully surprised by how Duke has handled all that has happened to him. I frankly could not have done it. He has been amazing. I think his connection with Pat Schafhauser has been great. Pat, as I mentioned, was paralyzed while playing professionally, and I think there has been a never-give-up connection with them.

Duke has said that he believes there is a reason, a purpose for all this. I don't know for sure. There are some religious aspects that go with those thoughts, and I go back and forth on them. I do know this:

whatever the reason, Duke has handled it, and handled it in the most positive way possible.

I don't know if coaching is in his future. I hear he is doing some things at Bowling Green, and that's great. When Duke was here, we had him involved with the team but not in the actual coaching area because we would not have been able to do that with him still in high school at the time. But here is the thing. If he got a college degree and wanted to be involved, and if he could show that he had a purpose that we could accept or even a borderline involvement, yeah, I would get him involved here with us.

I think Duke would also be good at motivating other kids through what happened to him. We did some speaking together at some young kids' hockey camps. We did it two summers in a row. I talked to the kids about what it means to be a high school player and Duke talked about, "You know you think you are this stud kid, and things can happen. You have to keep your windows and doors wide open to being a good kid. Treat people with respect and do the right thing." He brought some tears to their eyes.

Someone asked me once about Duke. I responded that he is an amazing kid. He is resilient. He sees himself as being the luckiest guy in the world. He is humbling to the rest of us. He has a great personality. He is funny and so entertaining. He is brutally honest.

I recall when he was here at the school recently and he said to me, "Hey Coach Lech, looks like you are losing a few of your head hairs. I can help you with that. I'll give you some of mine." And the kids who were here, some of my current players who heard it, I know they were thinking, *Oh, man, Duke, you can't be saying that to the coach.* And my thought was, *Yes he can. It's great!*

I love his genuine honesty. He is so caring and so professional in every way. I know he was sort of like that before, when he was younger, but now he has matured and is such a great positive and confident individual.

I also feel like it was amazing that after all he went through, he went away to school on his own. This is a kid who takes on new challenges all the time. He is such an inspiration to everyone who knows him. He has so much strength and so much passion that he will be a success in whatever he sets as his goals.

CHAPTER 7

Graduation

Six little words that are absolutely huge to me: I made it through high school. It wasn't easy—I won't lie about that. I had to have a lot of help along the way. My mom and dad were there for me and provided me with the support I needed. Hockey was over for me. There was never a question about that. So, too, were many of the other basics in life.

Getting my high school diploma and graduating with my class was a major goal for me. I was in the ninth grade when my world collapsed. Returning to school and life afterward, I had other priorities. Graduation was a high priority, but it seemed a long way away—especially if I were to tackle high school in the traditional sense. Attending regular school as I once had was not a viable option. There was no chance; I could barely function.

Instead, I was homeschooled for about two years, along with two to three therapy sessions a day. I'd go to several different places to get various kinds of treatment for my physical rehabilitation—working on things such as underwater treadmills to build up strength and coordination in my legs. I was in a wheel-chair, and basically starting over almost everything in life.

Even though I had been a student at Hill-Murray, we lived in the Edina school district. When it came time for me to restart my education, I began homeschooling. The local high school set the whole program up for me, sending teachers from the school with the same curriculum they taught to their students. Meanwhile, I had numerous infections in my brain that caused me to spend a lot of time at Gillette Hospital for rehab, and the teachers would come there, too.

I have to admit that it was a very difficult time for me because I got extremely tired from being physically worn out. It was very hard. Between school and physical therapy, I felt busy all the time. Still, on the positive side I kind of liked it because the athlete in me enjoyed hard work and conditioning. It became something that I sort of thrived on. I knew the hard tasks and constant activity would be good for my body. It also kept me continually occupied, so my mind didn't wander. It was physically and mentally challeng-ing, without a doubt.

During those years at home, it seemed like therapy, in addition to homeschool, was my whole life. I was in a wheelchair. I couldn't do anything. Hockey had once been my whole life and then sud-denly therapy had taken its place—a depressing thought. I was a mess, and I *had* to find a way to get better. I was especially upset about being confined to that wheelchair. I hated it, truly hated everything about it. Everywhere I went—with my mom to the store, to therapy, everywhere—I sat in that wheelchair. I tried to use it as little as possible. If I needed it, fine, but if not, I found a way to get out of it.

Strangely enough, I don't recall being angry during those therapy sessions. Sure, I was not happy about my situation, but in all honesty I remember feeling good being in those sessions because I was able to physically exert myself. Getting myself back to some kind of decent physical condition was important to me. And I enjoyed working at it. No, the therapy didn't bother me—in fact, I thought it was kind of awesome. As strange as it seems, the difficult workouts made me feel good.

I had some nurses who took care of me at home, and I really enjoyed being with them. They were like my buddies. So I had homeschooling, therapy, workouts, nurses; that was the sum total of my life at the time. There were a lot of people around and they all took care of me. I have always and will always appreciate it.

During this time, I had good days, bad days, and everything in between. This was one of the best: I was selected to ceremoniously drop the puck before a Minnesota Wild hockey game at the Excel Energy Center in St. Paul. Since the Wild franchise came into existence, there have only been eight individuals selected to drop the puck before a Wild game. Typically they are celebrities, great athletes—the Joe Mauer type, not a Duke Pieper.

To be asked to do such a thing was an incredible honor. I suppose they picked me because of all that happened to me. After all, I was a hockey player who had been hit by immeasurable tragedy. And the fact that people in the hockey world are so closely connected—well, I'm sure that had something to do with it.

I was being homeschooled at the time, so I didn't have much interaction with people outside my therapy sessions, so this was a really big boost for me. I really needed something like it to get my juices flowing and to really feel good about myself. I cannot express the honor I felt when my dad told me the team had asked for me to do this. All I can say when I think back on it is *wow*, even now.

The Wild had been great to me already. While I was in the hospital, the team had sent me all kinds of hockey gear and goodwill messages. So I felt like I had a great connection with the team from the beginning.

I was honored to drop the puck, but I was also anxious. The way it works is that before the game, the person selected comes out to center ice, joining the captains of the teams scheduled to play the game. Dropping the puck ceremoniously signals the beginning of play—kind of like throwing out the first pitch at a baseball game. I was asked to bring four of my Hill-Murray teammates with me for the event. I asked J.D. Cotroneo, Ben Bahe, Tim Shaughnessy, and Jack Walsh to join me. I had known J.D., Ben, and Tim for some time through junior hockey, and Jack was someone on the team that I just had a really good relationship with right from the start at Hill-Murray.

Luckily, I had seen this kind of event before during high school and college games, so I pretty much knew what to do. Which is lucky, because no one really gave me any instructions. Well, in reality, I suppose I was told in considerable detail what to do, but I was so focused on something else, I cannot recall a word of what I was told. That was the least of my worries.

There I was, about to walk out on the ice—and on a red carpet, mind you—to drop the puck in front of two great NHL players and more than 18,000 fans at the Excel Energy Center. Think about it. Me! I was standing out on the ice dropping the puck between Mikko Koivu of the Minnesota Wild and Rick Nash of the Columbus Blue Jackets—a dream come true.

To say I was nervous would be a colossal understatement. I

don't even know how to describe how I felt. I was terrified that I would screw the whole thing up. I wasn't worried that I would walk out at the wrong time, drop the puck before I was supposed to, or anything like that. No, I was frantically nervous because I did not want to fall down. I was afraid I might fall in front of all those people.

After all, I was no longer the flashy ninth-grader who had made the Hill-Murray varsity hockey team. The ice was no longer my comfort zone. My entire focus as I walked out on the ice with my four teammates was not to fall down, period. Remember, it hadn't been all that long since I had been paralyzed and couldn't eat, breathe on my own, or walk. I knew my balance was still off, and my walking was not all that great, so my anxiety was somewhat justified. So that was where all my concentration was on that wonderful night. Everything else was totally blocked out of my head.

Well, I didn't fall down. I was walking on the carpet and my teammates were right there with me, and I got to the center of the rink just fine. I recall looking at my feet, placing one foot before the other, one foot before the other. I didn't see it, but I was told before I came out on the ice and was introduced, that a story about me that had been filmed by Fox Sports North television played on the giant scoreboard above the rink. It was dark in the arena, there was music playing, and the 18,000 fans were cheering and giving me a standing ovation. I was wearing a Wild jersey with my old hockey number, and my teammates had their Hill-Murray jerseys on. It gives me chills to think about it today. It was great.

Once I got to the spot, I was able to relax a little bit. I knew something about how the puck was legitimately dropped during a game. It was something I had seen done thousands of times. I wouldn't say that I blew it or anything like that, but when I dropped the puck, I kind of dropped it toward the Wild captain, Mikko Koivu. Yep, I guess I did—right toward Mikko. It must have been because I love the Wild and I just couldn't help myself.

After, my friends and I went down to the locker room area and then later up to a special suite where we watched the game together. I received a Wild jersey autographed by the team. It was just a wonderful night, one I will never forget. The Wild were so nice to me and I am forever grateful to the organization for doing all they have for me. They wanted to make me feel special and they succeeded! It's something that I'll never forget.

I often think about that very special night. Think of it: 18,000 people cheering for you. It was really comforting to me that all those people cared enough to rise to their feet and clap their hands. It was an unbelievable feeling to see and hear all of them shouting for me. I had always dreamed about that moment—being on the NHL ice in front of a roaring crowd, but in another scenario. In that dream I was playing in a big game, scoring the winning goal, and the crowd was going wild. That would have been nice, too, but not the same feeling. When I dropped that puck, they recognized me for where I had come from and for where I was when I walked out on that ice. There are no words to describe what that meant to me, but I can say that it was more special than any game could have been.

It was an unbelievable experience, made even better by the fact that I got to meet Larry Hendrickson. Larry is an amazing man—and what a career he's had! He earned six letters in high school—three in football, three in hockey—and is in the Washburn High School Hall of Fame. He has done just about everything related to sports. He was the strength and conditioning coach at the University of Minnesota, served in the same capacity with

Herb Brooks' "Miracle on Ice" US Olympic Team, and later again with Herb with the Minnesota North Stars.

He also coached high school hockey at Benilde–St. Margaret's and was the state tournament runner-up while coaching at Richfield in 1976. He later coached the state championship team at Apple Valley in 1996. He was inducted into the Minnesota Hockey Association Coaches Hall of Fame in 2010. Hockey has been a lifelong passion for him. Retired from coaching, these days he is actively involved in promoting hockey for the disabled.

Larry is the father of current Minnesota Wild assistant coach Darby Hendrickson, who introduced us to each other. (Darby had been at the event that night representing Fox Sports North.) Larry and I hit it off immediately and remain close friends today. Even with my busy schedule, I try to keep in contact with him. When I am home, I try to get over to his house. He has a garage full of amazing workout equipment that I have enjoyed using on several occasions.

Even though I was in such dire straits physically, for the most part I did my best to be happy. Nights like that one in St. Paul sure helped. My goal was to try to get back to being a normal person again. After two years of what seemed like constant therapy and schooling, I had greatly improved. I had reached the 11th grade, and I was ready to return to traditional school. I was faced with a decision as to where I wanted to go. Edina was close to home, and I had been homeschooled by teachers from their system, but I had my heart set on attending Hill-Murray. I had been absent for almost two years, but I felt good there. I wanted to go back. I knew people there. I knew the teachers, the students; many were my friends. I had played freshman football there, too, which was also meaningful. In short, I loved the school, the setting and the surroundings. I was comfortable there. And with the condition I was in physically and mentally by the fall of 2011, I felt it was the place for me to be and to be able to look forward to high school graduation in the spring of 2013.

Hill-Murray was a known quantity. Edina, other than the handful of teachers I met, was a giant question mark. I was worried about whether I would be accepted there. The students wouldn't know me. Most of the teachers wouldn't know me. I didn't want to feel like everyone was looking at me thinking, *Who is this weird kid and what happened to him?*

During the time I was homeschooled, my mom did a great job keeping everything coordinated so that I could go back to Hill-Murray. Edina is a public school. Hill-Murray, on the other hand, is private, and the academic requirements are more rigid. This meant that the curricula weren't identical, and some of the classes I had taken through Edina teachers were not eligible for credits at Hill-Murray. Eventually the two schools worked it all out, despite a number of classes that weren't directly comparable. I am very thankful to all those involved that assisted in the "merger" so to speak. And I am very grateful for all that the Edina system did for me. They were spectacular.

I had a lot going on in my life, and, as I mentioned, one of the things that really helped me was to come in contact with Larry Hendrickson, who has had such a positive impact on my life. He helped me to stay positive, and to work toward my goals. Well, I stayed the course, and was able to enroll in Hill-Murray to begin my junior year. My first day back was exciting, but I was also really nervous. After all, I had been gone for almost two years. I was not the same physically, that was a given. Mentally, I felt that I was pretty strong. But without question, I was somewhat self-conscious about my disabilities and the way I looked. I had some facial distortions, and I definitely looked different than I had when most people last saw me. I was concerned about what people would think of me.

I don't think I did a very good job of keeping up with everyone from my past. Even though I wanted desperately to get back to Hill-Murray, all of it was going to be pretty new for me. I knew a lot of people from my freshman year and they knew me, but most of them hadn't seen me or been around me since then. Most didn't have the first clue what had happened to me or what I had been through.

I wasn't sure what to expect. I wasn't sure what they all would think of me. And actually, I never found out because I never asked them. But as far as I can tell, I felt like I was accepted very well. The reality is that there will always be some people who don't know what to say to you. Maybe they don't want to hurt your feelings, or they're just uncomfortable around you. That's okay. I have accepted that and understand why they might feel that way. Everyone is different in the way they handle things, and I can accept that. I don't hold anything against the people who feel uncomfortable around me or who choose to just ignore me. I do get it; I do understand.

For the most part, returning was a great experience. It was the right decision for me, even though it was quite a distance from home. I fit in almost right away and that meant a great deal to me. I had many significant accommodations where it came to class work, and the teachers were fantastic in helping me in every way possible. They were absolutely awesome. Whenever I needed anything, they were right there for me. Every time I made an effort to go and see them or needed anything, they were right there to help. And if they couldn't meet my needs they pointed me in the right direction toward getting what I needed. I cannot thank them enough.

One of the toughest classes I took when I returned was biology. It was a very difficult class, and if it wasn't for Mr. Paul Otto, it would have been even tougher for me. Mr. Otto was great and worked with me every step of the way. He also kept in contact with my parents through the school year. He is one of those special teachers who really made a mark on my life. I survived biology, and what's more, I got a friend out of the process.

I also reconnected with the hockey team right away. I was around the team all the time, got to chill out with the guys; I almost felt like I was on the team again. The coaches were terrific to me, too. They had kept in contact with me while I was going through everything and even came to visit me in the hospital a couple times, so they understood everything I had been through. That was important for me to have that shorthand with the coaches and team members. I felt like I was back on the team again, one of the members—just not a player.

For the most part, it was a pretty easy fit for me to return to the fold. I had been with the guys in the past, and that was one of the biggest reasons I wanted to return to Hill-Murray. I went to the games and attended practices. I had pasta night with the team. I felt like I was a part of hockey again. It was painful not to be playing, but it was the best I could hope for.

Not being able to play hockey with the team hurt a lot. My doctor initially had hope that in a couple years I might improve enough to play again, but that was wishful thinking. I knew that there was no possible way I was going to be able to play in the near future, and likely never again. Certainly not at the level I had been playing.

I have always tried to be honest with myself. I tell myself straight out, *Don't hide anything.* And I was brutally honest with myself during these times: *You are not going to play again.* Returning to high school, and a normal level of socialization, was good for me, but to be honest, it was also a very tough time. There were several occasions with the hockey team when I got to feeling pretty sorry for myself. *Why aren't I out there playing? Why me? WHY ME?* I guess that was pretty natural to feel that way, like an older player does looking back on his glory years. I just can't let that feeling go. Just recently, I was watching the state high school tournament with my dad and told him, "This really sucks. I should have been able to be out there, to play in the state tournament. It sucks!"

I mean, I had it all. I was a good player. Who knows what would have happened. How good would I have been? How good would our team have been with me? I missed out on playing in several state high school tournaments. That was supposed to be me. I was supposed to be there. And I never was. It was tough to think about that and still is to this day. But there is not one single thing that I can do about it, so I can't dwell on it. I cannot change a thing. It has passed me by.

One of the great traditions for the hockey team is Senior Night, and this unleashed some incredibly mixed emotions in me. Indeed, it is an emotional evening for all the players. It takes place before the final home game of the regular season and recognizes all the outgoing seniors. (Most sports teams have a similar event to show appreciation and acknowledge the players who are playing their final year.)

At Hill-Murray, it is kind of a big deal. The seniors are called out one at a time, and the players each go out on the ice with a bouquet of flowers, which he presents to his parents. After giving the flowers, the players and their respective parents then go across the ice together to the opposite side of the rink and receive applause and fan recognition. It is designed as both a thank-you to the parents and tribute to the players for their accomplishments.

I was a part of the team, so I was involved like the rest of the seniors. Not surprisingly, the only thing on my mind when taking the ice was not to fall down and make a spectacle of myself. I was so nervous. I had not been on skates in a game for almost three years. I had fooled around some with my skates on, but when I got on the ice, my ankles were so weak that I could barely stand up. This, combined with my other issues, like balance, made it very difficult. Two of my teammates helped me. One on each side of me, holding me up, we made it across the ice to my parents. I remember saying to my mom, "I am so nervous, you are going to have to hold me up." I was actually shaking. But we made it, and it was a very nice occasion.

As I reflect back, it was sometimes a difficult pill to swallow. In my bad moments, I think, *Here I was a gifted young hockey player, nationally recognized, making the varsity of a championship high school hockey team as a freshman. And then I am being helped across the ice in fear of falling.* Life can change quickly, and at the most unexpected times.

Yet at the time, such thoughts escaped me. My total attention was devoted to just getting across the ice in one piece. There were too many things going on around us, and I was only trying to get to my parents looking halfway normal. It worked out.

Being able to recognize my parents that night was a great opportunity for me. I cannot say enough how much I appreciate what my parents did for me through all those difficult times. I'm sure it was so hard for them. They gave up everything for me, and have always been there when I needed them. And they still are! To let them know how much I appreciated them in that moment, and in front of everyone else, was an honor.

As a parting shot, the team won second place in the state tournament. Even though I was not playing, I got to go out on the ice after the game and accept the trophy for the team. It was incredibly special. I had been named one of the team captains for the entire season. It was an exciting time being named team captain, and clearly a great honor. Earlier, when I came back to Hill-Murray, Coach Lechner had mentioned me being a captain. But a lot of time had passed since then and I had pretty much put it out of my mind. And then it happened. It was also special the way I found out. Coach Lechner did not tell me ahead of time. When he made the announcement to the team as to who was going to be the captains for that season, he just called off my name. It was extremely humbling. He had already done so much for me; to be named captain on top of it was a tremendous thrill for me and my family.

The captains had the honor of accepting the trophy for the team. It was a big deal, but I have to admit that at the time, again, all I could think about was not falling when I went out on the ice. Luckily, again, I didn't fall and that was a huge relief. I had my Hill-Murray jersey on and it was a great honor going out there on behalf of the guys.

Being one of the team captains was very special for me. It was incredible. I don't want to sound cocky or unappreciative but it was always my plan to be up there. From the ninth grade, I thought to myself, *Look, I am going to be one of the best players on my high school team. I am going to lead the team to the state tournament and I am going to be captain of that team.* It was just the way I thought. It really was. I had all the confidence in the world. So even though it was a little different scenario, being a team captain fit right into my expectations. Still, when it actually happened, it was a tremendous thrill.

To be a captain for that team was fantastic. Sure, it didn't happen the way I'd first imagined it would, but I think the way it turned out made it even more special and made me appreciate and respect it even more. I had a good relationship with the coaches and the players on the team, and it capped that final season beautifully.

Those high school days were filled with some exceptional moments as well as some tough times. As I look back, I realize that everything was not perfect, but then who *can* say that about their high school experience? The way my school and teachers handled my disabilities was incredible. They were awesome, and helped more than they will ever know.

Schoolwork was tough, I'm not going to lie about that. It is tough to go to class and try to learn with double vision. And my balance was a problem that I had to cope with every single day, too. So physically I had to deal with these issues (and, frankly, many more).

The real downer, of course, was not being able to play hockey. It was my dream, one of the major reasons why I was at Hill-Murray to begin with. So one might ask, "Why would you even want to go to school if your dream was taken away from you? What would the point be?" I mean, at one point in my life, the whole purpose of school was to play hockey, graduate, and then move to the college level and then the pro ranks. So why would I even want school without hockey?

Well, I learned different. I know there is a reason for all this, and eventually I will know what that reason is all about. I am confident about that and feel certain that my purpose will reveal itself. Maybe it is to help others, tell my story, write a book. Who knows for sure? I guess I will find out.

I committed all my energy toward the goal of graduating on time with my class. I went to summer school to accomplish that. I worked hard every single day. It wasn't easy. I am no genius. I was not gifted in the classroom, I know that for sure. But I finished. I am proud of myself for making it, considering all the extra issues I had going beyond the norm. I had a lot of help, and my mom is first in line for my gratitude. I would not have made it without her. It was such an important goal for me, and I completed it: I graduated with my class, on time. And you know what? Graduation was magnificent.

The ceremony was at the Cathedral of St. Paul. It was a great evening, the culmination of years of hard work. I recall walking up onstage to get my diploma. Even then, I was not able to take all the excitement and joy because I was keenly focused on making it up and down the stairs without falling. That was key for me. And I did, and it was just a perfect evening. I'm very proud of what I accomplished.

There with me that night were so many of my teachers who had helped me so much. They gave me an abundance of encouragement throughout the school years and were so happy for me. After the diploma ceremony was completed—on the mammoth indoor stage—we filed out of the St. Paul Cathedral, where all the teachers were lined up to greet each graduate. I felt really bad afterward because so many of them were talking to me and congratulating me, but I was giving all my attention to navigating the steps and not falling. I wish so much that I could have given each of them the attention and special thanks that they so deserved, but I have always been so grateful. I hope all my teachers know that.

I wish I had the ability to see what might have been. How would things have turned out if I had not suffered from brain issues? Would I have been a great player? How would I have played in the state tournament? How would my life have been different?

I know there is no point in focusing on those things. They will never be a reality, but I think it's okay to wonder about them once in a while, as long as I don't obsess about it. I wish things were different and had been different. But you know what? They aren't and they won't be.

There are nights when I think about it and just have a hard time. There is no cheering me up during those moments, and I have found about the only solution is time. But then I move on. I move ahead, and fight as hard as I can for some sort of normalcy in my life. That may be my biggest accomplishment yet.

Duke Is the Teacher

Paul Otto,
Hill-Murray Biology Teacher

I HADN'T KNOWN DUKE AT ALL BEFORE HE CAME BACK TO HILL-MURRAY for the 11th grade, though I had heard some about him and knew of the difficult time he had gone through. I am from Edina, so I felt like we had an initial connection.

The first thing that impressed me about Duke more than I could ever explain was that given all he had been through, he never showed it. He conducted himself as if nothing had happened to him. He acted as if nothing was wrong. He wanted nothing special, didn't want anyone to feel sorry for him, and just went about his business like everyone else. He was amazing.

Duke had a tough time but never asked for any kind of break. He wanted to be treated like everyone else. He was always open to anything. I knew from the beginning that he was going to be all right. I mean, how could he not be with the incredible attitude and passion for life that he possessed? His parents were also fantastic. They kept in communication with me and offered any and all support they could. I have great respect for them the way they offered to assist.

I only had Duke for one biology class, but he left an impression on me that will last a lifetime. He was so positive, so optimistic, never carried an ounce of self-pity, and was such a pleasure to be around every day.

I found he was so easy to communicate with in all aspects of my class. He was always respectful and incredibly personable. Biology is a tough subject, and Duke was a tremendously hard worker. He seemed like he just simply enjoyed every single day, and I found that he never gave anything but his very best.

Duke Pieper stands out among others. He gives his best and brings out the best in everyone around him. He is a fun person to know, fun to talk with when you see him, he brings out a smile in you. He is that kind of person.

High school is not an easy time for kids. There are a lot of pressures and a variety of issues to be coped with every day. I can't imagine how all this was for Duke given what he had been through and was continuing to go through. And yet you would never think there was a problem. His attitude was remarkable.

I have always felt that he is the epitome of taking what God has given you and then doing the best with it. Here is a kid who has had his life upset in the most significant ways, and yet he makes no excuses, feels no entitlement to anything, and just does what he needs to do. Tell him what to do and he will do it. He is that kind of person. The reality is, Duke is the teacher. He teaches us. He shows us the right way to be, the right way to conduct yourself, even under the most extreme circumstances.

I was not surprised to hear that Duke is in college and doing well. I never had a doubt regarding his success. And I'm glad he has written this book. He has a story to tell. His honesty and sincerity highlights every part of it.

Second to None

Pat Schafhauser
Assistant Hockey Coach, Hill-Murray

I KNEW OF DUKE A LITTLE BIT FROM THE COACHES, BUT I REALLY NEVER met him until he came to play for us as a freshman. I heard from others that he had the potential to be a pretty good player. The first time I saw him on the ice was during tryouts for that first season with us.

We had a good team, with most of our players returning from our state championship season, so I knew it was going to be hard for him or anyone new to make the varsity. Right from the beginning I realized that he had some skills. When you have been a player and been in the coaching ranks for a long time, you can sometimes tell right off the bat when a certain kid has a feel for the game. He showed us right away that he might be someone to keep an eye on, even as a younger player.

He was a good-sized kid, with good presence on the ice. We saw a confidence in him—actually, an extreme confidence—and that caught my attention as a coach. We had graduated a couple very good defensemen and had a spot or so available. The coach told me to take a little longer look at Duke even though he was only a freshman. We just saw something in him right away that stood out for us.

I watched Duke closely during camp, and it didn't take long for me to come to the conclusion that this kid was varsity material. The competition at Hill-Murray is quite intense, and usually older players show up better, so this was an unusual situation. We don't have all that many players as young as Duke perform so well. I could see early on that we were going to bring him right into our program and let him grow with it. I had a pretty good feeling that eventually, with some experience, he was going to be a special player for us.

That night in Burnsville was a night I will not forget. First, I want to go back about a week before the first regular-season game. We were playing at Cretin High School and I noticed a couple things happen that were unusual for Duke. During that scrimmage I watched him fan on a couple shots. I mean, this was not him just missing the puck but missing by quite a distance, maybe a foot or so. That was very unusual for Duke. I wasn't sure what to think about it at the time. I thought maybe he wasn't feeling well that night. Now, I didn't know (and still don't) if that was the beginning of something serious or what. I just know that I noticed something rather odd about those couple instances.

At the first game, I didn't notice anything unusual during warm-ups. He was a freshman, first-year player on the varsity, so I expected some nervousness, of course. When everyone came off the ice and entered the locker room, I can recall what happened next as if it occurred yesterday; it remains so clear to me.

Everyone was doing his thing before the game. Some were sitting by their lockers quietly, others were fixing their equipment, mostly just getting ready. Duke came over and said he was feeling kind of dizzy and not feeling well. Initially, I thought it was nerves, first-game jitters. I told him, "Don't worry about it. It's just nerves. Get a drink of water and sit down and you will be fine." Based on what he was telling me, I became concerned and was convinced he could not play. I wanted him to take his gear off and get in touch with his dad. I was concerned that it could be much more serious than initially anticipated. It was a day or two later before any of us learned the severity of what had happened to him and what he was facing. I can still see him standing there leaning over me and talking about how he was feeling at the time. It was a night I will never forget.

I went to see him in the hospital later on. In the beginning he could not have visitors, as he was in pretty bad shape. I remember entering his room and seeing a different person in the bed than I had known before. I had known this strong, healthy kid and now was seeing a young man, very ill.

I have to admit, because of what happened to me it was very difficult seeing Duke in the condition he was in. There was an absolute connection between us. Even though the medical issues are different between Duke and me, I can so closely relate to what happened to him. The biggest difference is that he was so much younger than I was when I had my injury. I recall it was Christmastime, and people around the hospital were trying to be somewhat festive, and there he was fighting for his life. It was very hard going in there to see him like that.

After his homeschooling, he came back to Hill-Murray and spent a lot of time around the team. I could not believe how he handled everything. I think he did so much better than most people could have imagined he would. From my own personal experience, I know it was hard to go back. You see everyone else doing things you would have been doing and it's hard to realize that the world keeps turning no matter what happens to you. Life moves on, and it is hard to accept. Duke was unbelievable, to say the least. It must have been very hard for him—and he did so well at school and with the team.

The team was great to Duke. He was welcomed back. And yet it was a real eye-opener for everyone. We saw his sense of humor come back, and he fit right in again. I watched him deal with everything on a daily basis, and even though he did so well, I honestly hurt for him. It was almost like he was trapped inside his body and could not do the things he wanted to do.

Duke Pieper is the toughest kid I have ever been around. He has a mental toughness and an emotional toughness second to none. He is amazing. For him to handle what he has had to handle at such a young age is incredible. He is so mature and was much more aware of things long before he needed to be. He is a special kid to be around. I love having him around here.

I was with him when he was trying to walk with the leg braces and the wheelchair. Those are very hard things to overcome. He deserves to have a book written about him. He has earned it, and has a story to tell others. I give motivational speeches like I know he wants to do at some point. I tell a story about me not always being like I am today. I talk about how life can hit you in the face, some to a greater extent than others, but everyone will have to deal with issues, and there will be choices to make about how you move along with life. Duke can do that, too.

Despite all that has happened to him, he is living his life. He went off to college at Bowling Green alone. I couldn't believe he chose to do that, and I have heard he is doing well. I'm not a single bit surprised. No doubt, he is living his life.

CHAPTER 8

Going It Alone

As I got close to finishing up what I needed to do to graduate, I actually started to focus my attention on finding the right fit for college. There was a time when college seemed out of reach for me, but I had worked hard to get there. Even more amazing, more of my attention was focused on finding the right college and not on my health. Still, my health problems remained, and were a considerable factor in choosing the right fit for me as an undergraduate.

There were so many colleges out there and so many possibilities for me that it was overwhelming. And even though my focus was off my health issues for the time being, they would definitely play a part in my ultimate selection. The first big decision for me and my family was whether I would go to college nearby or choose someplace out of state.

One might think at that time in my life, going to school away from home was not in the cards. After all, so many people helped me on a daily basis—how could I leave that comfort zone? I'm sure that most people who knew my situation assumed I would have to stay at home. I mean, who was going to take care of me if problems developed? Who would I go to for assistance if I was across the country? Traveling to a school and being away from home seemed more difficult, but it was definitely an option that both intrigued and excited me.

But old habits die hard. I had always imagined I would go away to school. This was a high priority for me before my illness, and it still remained something that was very important to me. The second-most-important thing was that I wanted the school I attended to be a Division I school with a hockey team.

Of course, my original goal was to go to the school on a hockey scholarship. It had been my dream to play Division I hockey. It didn't have to be a huge school necessarily, but definitely one of the top schools for the sport.

Another thing I envisioned was a campus-style institution. I could see myself walking on the campus to my classes. It just felt right to me, and I could still see myself in that environment despite the turn my life had taken. I wanted that kind of a collegiate atmosphere, but not at a school quite the size of the University of Minnesota. I always felt that UM was too big for me. I wanted a little smaller setting.

Even though the part of my dream that included skates, sticks, arenas, and championships as a player was gone, the template for my ideal school remained. My role in college would now be as a student first, but I hoped to be involved in its hockey program to some extent. It was the best that I was going to be able to do; I knew I couldn't ask for much more than that.

When I visited Bowling Green in Ohio, I felt there was just something special about the school and the people there. It made my decision, despite any reservations about being far away from home, an easy one to make. Bowling Green assistant coach Ty Eigner is from Eden Prairie, and he had become familiar with my situation. He followed it through all the media coverage, so he knew my story well. When he became their assistant hockey coach, it gave me somewhat of a connection to Bowling Green. Moreover, it was Coach Eigner who got me connected with the head coach to some extent.

I visited the school in July, before school started in the fall, and talked to the head hockey coach, Coach Bergeron, and the rest of his coaching staff. Coach Bergeron was great right off the bat. He said I could do anything I wanted to be involved with the team. He said I could even be out on the ice helping the team if that was something I wanted to do.

I really felt like it was going to be a good place for me to go to school. It wasn't a huge university like Minnesota, but it was a nice size at 20,000, with a real collegiate atmosphere. I liked the way it was laid out. It is a beautiful place, especially in the summer when it's truly gorgeous.

The other thing I needed to do was make sure it could meet my disability needs. Bowling Green was able to do that, and was committed to assisting me. For starters, it offered various services and devices that would help me to read, write, and do the basics in school. I would also be provided time extensions to complete assignments and other projects.

In addition, I had to find the right place to live. My dormitory needed to be close to my classrooms as well as the other school activities I would be involved in. The school met those needs also. I could not have been more appreciative of how the people at Bowling Green went out of their way to assist me. I knew from the get-go that Bowling Green was a special place.

July orientation was very difficult. It was almost too much. One of the first orders of business was a campus tour. I was with my mom and dad, and we were whisked to this place and that place, and over here and over there—it was close to being overwhelming. We were meeting people everywhere we went. I cannot even remember all the things we did, but it was a whirlwind. Still, I was sold. I loved the campus and all the arrangements that the school was willing to make for me.

In many respects, that campus visit was a double dose of reality for me. First of all, for any freshman, taking in all there is to take in on his new college campus for the first time is interesting, confusing, and overwhelming. It is a completely new experience for anyone. For me, that was certainly true, too, but my medical condition was an added dimension. The whole experience was all the more incredible, as well as more daunting. I mean, I was excited to take it all in, and I really liked what I saw, yet I couldn't help but wonder, was it going to be too much for me?

I don't think my reservations were so much physical as they were mental. It was like I wasn't sure that my brain was going to be able to cope with all that was going on. I don't know how the brain works, but I wasn't afraid it would go haywire or something. I just know it was a little too much for me in the beginning. In many ways, I lost the experience. I could not seem to grasp what I was seeing and observing. When it was over, I couldn't really say that I took anything away from it; it remains a blur to this day. Maybe that's how everyone feels on their first day; I don't know. But I did know that Bowling Green was the right place for me. It was where I wanted to go to college in the fall of 2012.

The best part of all turned out to be the meeting with Coach

Bergeron. And I told the coach that I would do anything to help the team. No one ever promised that I would be a student-coach or anything like that, but it kind of turned out that way. I do what they need and help out with some of the scouting—anything I can do to help.

I was on the precipice of a huge change. Orientation might have been a blur, but I was excited to be going to college and living far away from home for the first time (no, the hospital doesn't count!). I was really pleased that I could have a connection to the hockey team and also relieved that the school could meet my needs with regard to living accommodations.

I was excited about hockey. I wasn't going to play in any games, but I was going to be a part of the school and a part of the team. So it wasn't plan A, but what choices do you have in life? Just do the best you can. I was way past the idea of ever playing again; I had a different set of goals for my life.

Previously, my biggest goal was to have a long playing career in the National Hockey League. Today, it is all different. My dad asked me recently about my future, and there was no doubt in my answer that I want to stay around the game in some capacity. Ideally I would like to coach at some level. Just the thought of coaching makes me excited. Being an agent is another possibility. I also have an interest in motivational speaking.

When school started in the fall, everything seemed so new. Maybe it was because I didn't learn a thing during my orientation period, or maybe that's just the way it is for everyone. At any rate, it felt like a fresh start to life. I was excited. I had to figure out where I was going, what I was going to be doing, but that was part of the fun. I used a GPS phone app to help me get situated, and that helped somewhat. It helped me locate landmarks, buildings, and classrooms on campus. That was a lifesaver for me, especially during my first weeks and months there.

Bowling Green State University is located in the town of Bowling Green, Ohio, which is about 20 minutes south of Toledo and about an hour south of Detroit, Michigan. Its campus sprawls over more than 1,000 green and hilly acres. It evokes such a great feeling in me, the feeling that you want to be there. You want to walk across campus to your classes. You want to go out and just lie on the grass and enjoy the day. It is an inspirational place, a place I really enjoyed from my first day. It fits the bill for me.

The weather at Bowling Green tends to be very windy, so it is a little different from what I am used to in Minnesota. I love walking around the campus to my classes or going to the ice arena. The setting is so pleasant and so conducive to learning. Sometimes I have to walk a fair distance to my classes, but that's fine. I love to walk, and am always grateful for the exercise. It works out well.

The ice arena kind of reminds me of Aldrich Arena in the Twin Cities, and indeed they are somewhat similar. It is a little small and shared by the student body and the community. It also has offices for some of the other athletics programs' coaches. It is a good hockey building.

From the outset, college presented some pretty large impediments. For one thing, I was going to attend college out of state—away from my comfort zone, my friends, relatives, and family. I didn't know anyone at Bowling Green. How were they going to look at me? Would they accept me? What were people going to think? I didn't know, and it was kind of intimidating for me.

This was an extra burden on top of everything else that comes with being a freshman. The new setting, so different from high school, was enough in and of itself. There were so many unknowns.

But for me I had additional anxieties about how I would make connections with my fellow students. At Hill-Murray, I had reintegrated into a student body where I was known before my accident. *Will I be able to make new friends?* I wondered. *Will the way I look bother people? Will I always wonder if people are scrutinizing me?* Those were some big fears to take with me to college along with the regular anxieties. And to be completely honest, it was much tougher than I ever thought it would be. But I had to keep reminding myself, it was nothing compared to what I had already gone through—and survived.

I have learned some things about first impressions. I know that people form an impression of someone rather quickly. Naturally, I wondered what people's knee-jerk impression of me would be. On campus, I didn't know anyone. No one had read my story. No one knew what happened to me and what I had gone through.

When I look in the mirror and see myself, I have a clear impression of who I am. And I hope that when people look at me, they think this way: *Hey, here is a kid that has been through a lot. What he has gone through, I don't know, but he's been through something. He wants to just be a normal kid, do what others do. He wants to be a normal person even though he is not. He may do things a little differently, but he will get them done. He wants to read a book like everyone else. He wants to play a game like everyone else. And he will, just in a different manner.* I hope that people will think about me that way when they look at me.

I can't do things the same way that others do, but I still want to fit in. I want to belong, and I will find a way to get things done and be as normal as possible. But I am different, at least bodily. My eyes are different; I see double. I have trouble with hand-eye coordination. My depth perception is off. My balance is off too, because my right arm is stronger than my left arm and my left leg is stronger than my right leg. My right hand used to be my dominant hand, but now it is not as strong or coordinated. My walking is different because I had to learn it all over again. I guess I don't put my feet down the way a normal person does, or at least the way I used to. But these are physical things. I think I am normal. What you see on the surface isn't all of me.

I recall that on my first day of college we had to stay in a hotel because the dorm was not ready. I was standing in the lobby of the hotel, listening to this lady who was addressing a group of us. While I was standing there in the lobby listening, a man came up to the side of me and asked me if I was okay. I hadn't done anything. I wasn't falling down, losing my balance, or anything like that; I was just standing there. My illness has caused me to have some facial deformities, and I guess he thought that because of the way I looked, there must be something wrong with me. He must have thought I needed help. The whole scene was kind of dramatic and I didn't quite know how to react to it. I told the man, "No, I'm fine. I'm just standing here waiting for the lady to get done talking to us."

I know that because of what happened to me I am now different. I look different. But you know what? That's okay, because I am still *me*. I'm still Duke Pieper. I think the same and am the same person.

I know I look a little different from others and I act differently than some, too. A couple people have asked me what happened to me. I am somewhat uncomfortable talking about my medical issues with people, but I try to be honest. I told some I was injured while playing hockey, have had many complications, and more than 10 different surgeries that have left me with several disabilities. I told them that one of the surgeries left me with a couple months of paralysis. I told them that this required me to learn everything again, including walking, talking, eating, breathing, and so forth. I suspect that response overwhelmed my listeners but was an ice-breaker to some extent. I know that most people, when they hear this kind of thing, cannot imagine anything even remotely like that ever happening to them. It is so far out there and there is such a remote chance of it that it does not even sink in to hear about it. I would have been that way, too, if the shoe were on the other foot. The difference is, it *did* happen to me.

I think after I told my story, many of the guys who I was starting to hang out with felt for me, and for the most part tried to understand. However, some of them were more like, "Don't bother me with that stuff." They don't care, and that's okay. That's life.

I knew from the start that making friends was going to take a little while; I was pretty sure of that. I tried to get myself out there with others as much as I could, but at first I wasn't having much luck meeting the type of people I wanted to meet. I felt somewhat lost in the beginning. My dorm was filled with not only freshmen but many upperclassmen, and they already had their friends.

After a while, I changed to an all-freshman dorm and that made it a little easier. But it wasn't all wonderful. It wasn't easy for me to make connections at first. For the most part I was feeling pretty good, but the newness of everything was very overwhelming for me. Once I got situated with the hockey team, it broke some barriers. The hockey guys made it much easier. Back in July, I was kind of introduced by the coach as someone who was going to be helping. When fall came, he reintroduced me to the team. That really meant a lot to me.

Socially, I think I am doing well. I have not been excluded. I go to class and I am involved in helping out with the hockey team. It might have been difficult to feel a sense of belonging without a team to be around, but I've been lucky in that respect. My hockey friends and the team atmosphere with players, coaches, and staff have really helped me to fit in and find my niche at Bowling Green.

Coach Bergeron has been really good to me. But I understand the pressures that go along with coaching at a big-time school, so I try to avoid being any kind of distraction for him. I'm around. I hang out. I watch practices and games and sometimes I attend team meetings. I have been accepted very well by the team and the staff, and I appreciate it so much.

Another one of the things I have tried to do to integrate into the Bowling Green community is to become acquainted with the local church. God has always played a big role in my life. I was raised Lutheran; my family attended church most Sundays. I was baptized and confirmed. While at Shattuck–St. Mary's, students were required to go to church, so I was pretty consistent there.

My faith has always been there, though I never was the type that paid a lot of attention to it. I just kind of went with the flow of going to church—it was something I did—but prayer never was a mind-centering thing for me. I went to church on Sunday and that was kind of it until the next week. I would get out of service and go do whatever I did.

It wasn't until my life-changing experience that the connection came into focus. In the beginning, as I mentioned, I was really angry with God. What I had learned in church had been mostly good things—how God was good to people who believed. Then suddenly this thing, this horrible thing, happened to me. I would ask myself, *Where was God when this happened? Why didn't he take care of me and prevent all this? Where was he when I needed him?* I was hurt and scared and looking for someone to blame, so I took it out on God and everybody else. *My life was in a great place and now it is all screwed up, so what is the point of all this?* I would ask myself. I was really angry.

During this time period, especially when I was at my worst physically, I was seeing all kinds of therapists and psychologists whose charge was to get my mind right and get me through all that was happening to me from a mental standpoint. That used to really frustrate me and make me just furious, the thought of someone trying to adjust my attitude for me.

I'd be sitting there in those sessions, wondering to myself as they talked to me, *You don't know anything about me. You are not in my situation, you have never been in my situation, and you never will be in my situation. So how do you think you can help me, exactly?* They were trying in earnest to counsel me and guide my mind in the right direction, but it wasn't getting through. I never actually verbalized what I was thinking because I was trying to be respectful, but I went on thinking it all the same. I was miserable, and nothing anyone could have said would have helped.

I understand what they were trying to do, but it didn't work. Their job was to get my thinking going in the right direction, but I was beyond resistant. I knew I had to do it myself. So I decided I was going to get through it on my own—with one very big exception. I reached out and asked God for assistance. I wanted to build up a better relationship with Him. I felt as though it was important to eliminate the anger I had for God and get Him back in my corner. We were starting from rock bottom, but you know what? The good thing about rock bottom is that there's nowhere to go but up.

I went to church, started reading the Bible, and did some serious praying. Talking with God helped, and I started to feel better. This probably started around the point when I was home and started to be homeschooled. My life was in shambles. I didn't have much to look forward to, or at least I thought so at the time. I knew I was in trouble, and I felt it was time to reach out. *Why not give it a shot?* I asked myself. I was desperate to find a solution to my misery.

We had a discussion. I said to God, "I am going to give this a try. I am going to give 100 percent to get better, to come back to some kind of a normal existence. I am going to take advantage of everything at my disposal and I am going to try to make my life better. I cannot give up. I have to try to make the best effort possible to get better. I am going to give this a shot. I want to improve my walking, my talking—basically everything I have lost. Will you please help me? Will you be with me along the way?" I felt I had to appeal to God because I had absolutely no confidence in the specialists who were trying to mentally improve me. I knew this had to be me doing it with the help of God, and I am so glad we had this conversation.

The results speak for themselves. I am here today and far better off. I have improved by leaps and bounds, but I still have a lot ahead. God and I are a good team because I know He knows and I know He understands.

My relationship with religion and God is very important to me. When I am home in Minnesota, I go to church and I feel good about it. I have not joined any particular church at Bowling Green, but I have attended various churches around campus. I try to attend pretty regularly. Overall, I'm pleased about my new direction and I give credit to my connection with God. He has played a huge part in my life. He has been there with me during my darkest times. It took me a while to realize this, but I now know that I had help from a higher power in getting through those difficult periods.

I would never say what happened to me was a good thing. But, as I have said, I have learned so much. Not least of which is that what I have experienced has opened up my eyes to life and to people. It has given me a better perspective on the big picture: what is really important and what is just trivial. That part of all this, I can honestly say, has been a blessing.

Telling my story is difficult, but I do believe that it is an essential part of God's plan for me. I'm still learning how to do that. There was a time a while back when I gave a speech to some Minnesota hockey players who were competing to be on a national team. I was really nervous, and I'm not sure that it went very well. I think most of them knew who I was because of the publicity I got in the local press, but I wasn't happy with the results of my speech. I just didn't think it went so well. It wasn't terrible, but I thought afterward that I could have done a lot better.

At our Hill-Murray hockey banquet, I gave another short talk; that one went a little better. My goal is to keep on improving with every talk. Eventually, I want to speak to groups as a motivational speaker. I want to share my story because it is unique, it is unlikely, and it can help others through the trials they face in their own lives, whether they are similar or not.

I think people need to hear the "never give up" stuff, because sometimes in the midst of a struggle you can feel like you're all alone, like no one has suffered like you're suffering now. I know when I was at my worst times, paralyzed, unable to do anything, I was convinced no one really understood what I was going through. I did feel alone and struggled believing I was going to have to fight by myself. Feeling so alone like that can be pretty powerful stuff.

But I have never given up and I never will. Even in my lowest, darkest moments, it was my attitude that kept me going and got me through. I am a fighter! I have no problem working harder than ever to accomplish my goals. I'm not ashamed to ask for certain accommodations so I can succeed in school. I know I am different and that I need some assistance. I am okay with that aspect of my life.

I have a sheet that lists my disability needs, and I carried it with me to all my classes when I started at Bowling Green. I wanted to make sure that my professors knew what I needed to do well in my classes. Some of them want to know what happened to me so that they can best work with me, and that's okay. Across the board, my professors have been extremely helpful in meeting my needs. Initially I was involved in a writing course, a sports management course, and a speech communications class. It was all new to me, as it is for all new freshmen, but I had additional complications, obviously. Still, I suppose I share the same frustrations as any new college student. Who among us could be prepared for the college academic setting?

The accommodations provided by the school are terrific. Everyone has been so incredibly helpful. I hold my own in the process. If an instructor asks me a question in class, I usually do fine. If I have a quick second for a thought, it usually comes to me right away and I am for the most part correct with my answers. I can participate in class like everyone else. Where the problems come for me is when I have to literally take the time to think about things, an answer, a problem. For some reason when I am put in that kind of situation, I can become confused easily. I don't know why, but I do.

Early on I took a lot of the general classes, as do all freshmen and sophomores. Later I would be able to take the specialized classes connected to my major and minor. So far I have enjoyed all my classes—even the basics like writing, English, and business. I work hard at it, and one of my goals at Bowling Green is to maintain a 3.0 GPA.

The class I had the most trouble with was economics. For some reason, it proved to be very difficult. Then again, there was some reason for this. In the majority of my other classes, because of my disabilities and the accommodations that have been granted to me, I have access to the instructors' lecture notes. In econ, however, because of the format of instruction by the teacher, I did not. Instead, I had to rely on another student for the notes; that proved to be more difficult for me. I'm not taking anything away from that professor, or the student who assisted me. It just was not as easy by way of this method. I made it through, but it was definitely more challenging than my other courses.

I ended up doing quite well my freshman year. My most frustrating time came when I experienced some pressure in my head somehow related to my illness. I didn't know quite what it was. At first I thought it might be some kind of infection, and my biggest worry was that I might have to come home.

We found out through an MRI that I have a dislocated disk in my neck that may have caused some of the pressure. The doctor said that the stress of college life and upcoming finals may have been a contributor as well. He told me that these kinds of things would happen to me from time to time, so I shouldn't be surprised if it occurred again. It was really a stressful time, but it worked out that I was able to stay and finish up the second semester.

Finishing up my first year at college, I admit that I went about it a little differently from my fellow students. Nothing came easy for me. I had help. For example, most kids can write a paper, take down notes in class. I can't write a paper by typing it with my own hands, or jot down notes in class. I can do it on a computer, but not like everyone else. I do things my own way, but the important thing is that I do them.

Taking tests is another complicated thing. I need more time to get the work done. It works, but again, it's different from how the rest of the students do it. It takes me longer to process the questions and come up with the answers. Sometimes professors have short, timed quizzes in class. That type of thing is really hard for me because I need more time to think things through. Sometimes it is worth asking for more time; other times, I just do the best I can within the time constraints and move on.

I can't write at length, so I use a scribe whenever I take a test. A person will accompany me to the testing room and I will tell them what to write out. This is one of my testing accommodations. I have to be in a quiet area and usually have to read the questions out loud to kind of talk my way through them. Obviously, in a room with other test-taking students, I could not do that. Additionally, I cannot read well because of my double vision, so at times I have to have someone read the tests to me.

When I take a test, I always need more time than is typically allotted. Sometimes the length of time I need for assignments remains the same. I just need ample time to process things. As I said, the professors have been great at helping me in get the work done and fulfill my responsibilities with each class. I am very clear on one thing: I don't want any special favors. I want to earn my keep, so to speak. If I get a good grade in a class, I want to have earned the grade by turning in the work, taking the tests like everyone else, and being scored the way others are scored. I don't want anyone feeling sorry for me and saying, "Oh, Duke needs extra help so we will just give him a good grade." No way will I *ever* accept anything like that from anyone.

However, I do accept that I am different in a way that is not my fault. I know that I need some extra help and some extra time, but that is *only* to get me on a level playing field with everyone else. Once I am on that equal playing field, let the competition begin. That competitive fire will always be in me. I want to excel in the classroom just like everyone else. I think that's fair.

The biggest thing for me is that I am doing it. From an early age I had very solid goals in my mind about what I wanted for college. I made up my mind I was going to still accomplish those goals. Although it has not been easy, I am working my way through it. It is well worth it.

I haven't declared a major yet, but I am pretty set on choosing sports management, with a minor in entrepreneurship. Those areas seem to fit me and my career goals as I look to my future.

Day to day, things are good. I know some people may wonder things like, *How does this guy ever have a good day? He had his life pulled out from under him. Now he is supposed to go on living and have good days?* But I do. I keep moving forward, not looking back.

I have typical days like everyone else. One might look like this: I get up in the morning, take a shower, have some breakfast, then head out for the day. I usually walk over to the hockey arena and hang out for a little while. I might look at some game film; often the coaches will have something they'd like me to do or get involved in. This makes mornings something to look forward to. Even in the off-season, I remain involved with the team.

Most of my classes start late in the morning, and generally I have two in a row. I've been lucky in that I have been able to register for my classes somewhat early because of my disabilities, so I can choose my ideal schedule. I really like the idea of late-morning classes because that gives me time in the mornings for hockey and still leaves me with late-afternoon time for myself. Later in the day, I try to always get a workout in before turning to my homework. Typically, I'm done with everything I have to do by suppertime, so I have some free time in the evening.

Honestly I love everything about Bowling Green. I have good days there, and often great days. I am comfortable with myself and my recuperation. I have gotten to know my body and what I can and cannot do. I know what I still have to work on and how to compensate. I know the tests in school are difficult for me, but with the time that I am allowed, I have excelled. All told, I do extremely well with the playing field leveled.

I truly believe that each and every day I move closer and closer to normalcy. Most of my past frustrations are gone. I have accepted what has happened to me. It is so important not to dwell on the past but to move on to the future. I work very hard not to get bogged down with some of the things that are out of my control. Writing is a good example. I might be able to handwrite only a paragraph at a time. I'm slow, and I have trouble forming the letters. I'll get better eventually, but I know this will take more time. So for now, I compensate. When it is suitable and effective, I use a computer. If there is not a hurry to take notes or a test, I can use the computer and it works out fine.

As I've mentioned, looking back very rarely serves a purpose. Why would I want to do that? It only brings me pain. There *are* times, though, when I use my memories (or lack thereof) as a form of motivation. To demonstrate to myself how far I have come. I realize the accommodations that I have in school are necessary and fair, therefore they bring me no frustration—quite the opposite, in fact. Considering where I was, it is wonderful to be in school at all, to take tests, participate in class, and get good grades.

Consider this, for example. I recall the wheelchair days, and my first walking day—or better said, the first *attempted* walking day. I was hoisted out of bed with a lift and placed in the chair. The pain was beyond words. I was pushed around the floor for a brief time before I was overcome; it was too much for me. I got sick and the pain was unbearable. I insisted on ending the nightmare. I wanted to stop, give up, never get in that chair again. It was overwhelming.

I couldn't do a thing for myself. Someone even had to hold my head up because my neck muscles were totally shot from all the neck surgeries I had undergone. Later, during my first real walk-ing experience, it took two people to hold me up while I braced myself on the handle of a walking treadmill. I couldn't help but think about how different it was from effortlessly skating around a hockey rink. I had been in the hospital bed for so long that I had no strength. I could do nothing! *Nothing!*

Those memories remind me that I have come a long way. I am thankful to be where I am today. I keep putting one foot ahead of the other, knowing I still have a long way to go. But I am proud of what I have accomplished. After all, I am going to college on my own in the state of Ohio. It's a long way literally and figuratively.

I do not want this to sound cocky, but in some ways I feel good that I have put people to shame in some respects. There have been many people—medical personnel, friends, family, or just casual onlookers—who have said, "There is no way Duke will ever be able to do [blank] again." Fill in the blanks: walk, go to school, leave home…the list goes on. There have been a lot of skeptics out there about my progress, my future. And I have proved them all wrong. That makes me feel good. Don't get me wrong—I don't want to rub it in their faces. But I have had to overcome what many thought would be the impossible, including medical professionals who have seen similar situations in their own practices. So how *did* I defy those expectations? That's easy: by hard work. Easy to say, but hard to do. But I sincerely mean uncompromising, never-give-in, never-give-up, painfully hard work. And the payoff has been a magnificent reward. I'm very contented in my life these days.

I have so many things on my plate every day to get past. I'm not complaining, but have learned to cope with the many daily problems with which I am confronted. And that's okay. I do it without questioning it. It's my reality, and it will be from now on. I can't play hockey. I can't go out and throw a football around or play catch on a nice day. I can't study or take tests like a typical student. I will say this, though. I honestly believe that someday I will be able to do many of the things I used to enjoy. Riding a bike is one. My balance is off, so that's out of the question for me now. But I do think someday I will be able to get on a bike again.

There were so many people who said I would never get on skates again, but I have proved them wrong. I have been able to get on the ice and move slowly around a rink a little bit. Holding the stick and shooting the puck around a little is really tough, but I have been able to manage it to some extent. There won't be any scouts looking at me and I won't be on an organized collegiate team, but it's a start. It is actually pretty frustrating not to be able to do all the things on the ice that I used to do, but I have patience, I really do. Someday.

It truly sucks that I can't do what I used to do. And it sucks, too, to talk about or think about it. I got into a conversation one day with a friend about just this subject. I don't know why I ever engaged in the discussion, because as we got into it more, it became almost too painful to bear. I could not hold back the tears as we continued talking. It was almost as if a dam had suddenly collapsed. It hurt desperately at the time, but in the end I was glad it happened because it got things out in the open. And more than ever reemphasized for me how much I hate the word *can't*.

Here is the thing. *Can't* is not a word I ever use. It is so hard to think about what I "can't" do because it is not a word in my vocabulary. I try to stay away from the word and its meaning. Talking about *can't* leads to nothing productive. And there is not enough time for me to focus on the negative. I have too many things to do to waste my time. So I don't do it, period. Instead, I go the route of the positive: thinking about what I can do, what I can achieve if I put my mind and energy into it. I know it is much better to think that way.

Another thing that really works for me is to take on something that is doubtful in the eyes of others. If someone thinks I cannot do something, I will do everything in my power to prove them wrong. It almost feels like a dare. Driving a car is a great example. I can't tell you how many people thought I'd never do that again. Finishing college—that will be a huge one. That's just the way I am made. That's me, Duke Pieper: a competitor until the end.

My first year at college went well. I made some great friends. And I had a 3.0 grade-point average my first year, so I am really proud of what I have accomplished. When I look back on things, I know that I did okay. Even so, I know that I can do better and I will be working toward that goal. I have a long way to go.

Based on what I have accomplished, I am on track. At times, it is a grind—I won't lie about that. It's not fun to work so hard at everything day in and day out, but I know that if I stick with it, things will work out in the end. They always do. And the rewards that can come are incredible. I know this and have experienced it firsthand. I am confident that I will continue on the road to success. I am off to a good start so far. And when my journey is complete, when I get everything accomplished in school and life to meet my goals, that will be a time when I can say, "Duke, you did it. You beat the odds." But not yet. I'm just getting started.

We Are the Fortunate Ones

Chris Bergeron
Head Hockey Coach, Bowling Green State University

DUKE HAS BEEN AROUND THE TEAM NOW FOR ALMOST TWO YEARS. I feel like I get to know him a little better each time we come in contact. I know we have a good relationship, and I also have connected well with Duke's parents.

The one thing right up front that I can honestly say about Duke Pieper and his involvement with the Bowling Green hockey team is that he wants no special favors or any kind of special treatment because of what happened to him. I am so incredibly impressed by his independence and his wanting to stand on his own and not be treated differently from anyone else.

We have him involved with the team mostly by assisting us on the recruiting end. He does a lot of organizational things for us as we try to pick and choose which high school kids are going to be a good fit here. We get sent all kinds of things—tapes, DVDs, news clippings—and Duke helps us with keeping things on track and organized. This is huge for us.

Knowing Duke, he will do anything we ask, but never tries to insert himself into things. He is never pushy and only wants to do what we want him to do. And he does a great job for us. He attends team meetings, goes to practices, and is a part of the team just like everyone else. At this point he has not traveled with us yet, but I am hoping in the future we can make that a reality for him, too.

The main thing that stands out when you are around Duke is his positive attitude. He has had and still has so many challenges in his life and has had to persevere to a level few of us will ever be able to understand. And he does so with such a great attitude, always. His attitude, perseverance, independence, and spirit are unbelievable and make me very proud of him and proud to know him.

He gets along exceptionally well with the other players on our team. He just wants to be one of the guys. It's kind of like, "Just like me and be around me because I am Duke. Nothing more, nothing less."

He is around every single day and sets such a great example for others who have not suffered his kind of misfortune. He is a part of our team like everyone else, as I mentioned, but it is so much more than that.

I'm sure some might look at his connection to the team and think, *Gee, isn't it nice what the hockey team is doing for Duke, letting him hang around the team?* Well, let me say this: It is not like that at all. *We* are the fortunate ones to have Duke in our program. He does more for us than we could ever do for him. He shows us how to treat people, how to act, how to be professional. We have given him an open door, but the fact is he means a great deal to us. He is a remarkable young man, and I can assure anyone of the fact that the Bowling Green hockey program is better because Duke Pieper is a part of it.

CHAPTER 9

I Will Never Give Up

When I was younger, I made a promise to myself and so far I have kept it: I will never give up on the things in life that I want to accomplish. I'm not sure exactly when I made that commitment to myself, but certainly I had no clue what I was going to be facing in my life. Still, that pledge has remained through it all. *I will never give up! I will never let the barricades in life get in my way! I will fight through all roadblocks, whatever settles in my path!*

The promise was born from the thought that when I get older, I never want to look back on my life and see that I did not strive for the things that were important to me. I never want that to happen. I want always to be able to say at the end of the day, when I look back on my life, that I did the best I possibly could.

I accept the fact that I may not meet every single goal in life to the fullest extent, but I choose to control my own part in that. The way I see it, never giving up is giving it your best shot, your maximum effort. And I have and will continue to do that. That attitude is ingrained in me; it is simply the way I think.

I suppose I was in my early teens when I first made this commitment to my own success. Maybe it started during my early days at Hill-Murray, when I was going through tryouts. I remember we had a total of five tryouts that came back-to-back. The first two were just awful for me. For whatever reason, I really messed them up. I had made bad passes and done just about everything wrong on the ice that was possible to do. Worse, I was fully drained of energy. I had been putting so much effort into those practices that I had virtually nothing left—and yet the results were terrible.

Despite the dismal showing in the initial tryouts, I was able to turn it around. The last three sessions were better, and I think the coach saw the effort I put forth and that was the reason I made the team. And I didn't let up. I gave him my all each and every day in practices and games. As important as my talents on the ice were, my persistence and commitment to success were just as crucial.

Years later, after my injury, I remember sitting in an eye doctor's office waiting for my appointment. There was another guy, an attorney, waiting too. He overheard me complaining to my mom and kind of butted in to our discussion.

I was upset about something that had happened in the Edina system after I transferred there. I had to enroll in a particular class there even though I had taken a similar class at another school. I felt I should have been given the credit, but the school thought otherwise. I was really upset about it. The man listened carefully to what I had to say and then said to me, "You know, dude, you just have to get it done. Look, even though it is going to be a bitch to take the class over, just do it. Don't think about it, just do it. Get it done with and get it over with and then you are done with it."

His message really struck a nerve with me. *Just do it. Get it done. Don't waste your time and energy on something that you cannot control.* It was the right thing to hear at the right time. And I've never forgotten it.

After my brain injuries, this pledge to myself became a promise of a different magnitude. It is easy to say you will never give up in a hockey tryout or a class in school. That's easy stuff. But what about being paralyzed, thinking you may die, and starting over in learning even basic motor skills? Try that on for size. How does your "never give up" approach look now?

There were so many things I had to learn all over again. The easiest way to say it is that I had to learn everything, and that's only a slight overstatement. The list included walking, running, balancing, breathing, eating, drinking, swallowing, writing... I could go on and on. I recall trying to do things that kids might do in preschool. Coloring was one of those things I couldn't master initially. I remember trying to color between the lines, and I just could not make it happen.

Swallowing, eating, and drinking were complicated to learn, but they had a system in place in the hospital. It was tricky because the staff that worked with me had to be sure that the food would go down properly. They started by giving me slippery foods, like noodles with olive oil, that kind of stuff. There was a time when I had a feeding tube in my nose through which I was fed blended foods and liquids. That was terrible—I mean, absolutely *awful*. I had so many troubles during that time, I honestly don't know how I got through them all. And just when I would think, *This is as bad as it gets*, it got worse. I remember in the earliest days my dad would sneak me in Gatorade sometimes. He was not supposed to do that but he did anyway, and I really enjoyed it. At that time, eating normally was out of the question; all I got to do was eat some ice chips. Through the weeks and months, the hospital staff worked with me on it to keep my nutrition intact. At times I became overcome by emotion; I just could not believe what was happening to me. Was this nightmare just that: a nightmare? Or was this whole thing real? I answered the question quickly. It was real.

My paralysis was the cause of all the physical setbacks. Sitting in a hospital bed for so long, my muscles atrophied to the point where they were basically gone. I had to build up strength in most part of my body in order to function. So we took things incrementally, learning how to breathe and swallow, and then working up to things like walking.

No matter how bad things got for me, I know I kept the attitude of "I will never give up." But it was hard, every single day. I was a high school hockey player, and suddenly I would look at a coloring book page and think to myself, *A preschool kid could do a better job than this*. At times it seemed impossible to believe. There was no question I had a long way to go.

Through my recovery, I knew I just had to keep on learning. I had to get past the coloring and move on other things. There were many times I used to just stop everything and wonder to myself, *How am I going to do all these things that used to come so naturally for me? How am I going to walk, run again, play sports, or do anything close to what I used to do? If I can't even color inside a line, how am I going to survive all this?* There were some really depressing times when I couldn't help but become discouraged.

But I tried to focus on the big picture. I echoed what the man in the doctor's office said about putting my head down and getting it done. Those words, heard through complete happenstance, helped me through a lot of tough times. No matter how difficult or arduous something is in the moment, you have to find a way to get through it. *Just do it.* If it happens slowly, but there is a little improvement each day, that's okay. Get through it and do it. Don't give up.

I had to do the little things before I could get to the big ones. I had to color inside the lines. I could have protested, said "This is stupid" and walked away, but I didn't. I had to walk a line over and over to work to get my balance back. I could have chucked it all and refused to do it, but I wouldn't give up.

Working on getting my muscles to respond properly for all sorts of basic motor functions was difficult. It involved small exercises done repeatedly, or what seemed endlessly. Keeping a good attitude was really important because there were so many times when I had to fight to keep from total despair. For instance, I had a face-stimulation machine that I used to try to get the muscles working again. It delivered some type of electrical current that "woke up" the muscles and nerves in my face. I had to hold the pad to my face for about 15 minutes each day. I absolutely *hated* it…but I knew that it was important, so I did it.

As I got better, I was able to exercise somewhat. Even when I was able to do very little, it helped me. It kept my mind right, kept up my spirit. I have always been the type of person to keep myself in good shape. That mentality has obviously been helpful in my recovery. I don't like to run, but I force myself to do it because the results are hard to argue. I still enjoy working out, yet I am uncomfortable being around others while doing it, so it's been difficult for me to be in gyms and other settings like that. Hockey provided the initial impetus for me to start working out and get in good shape. My workouts are far different from what they used to be, but I have come a long way from where I began after the injury.

I take great pains to work out the right way. It has always been kind of bothersome to me that people spend the time to work out but don't really know what they are doing. I don't mean to say I am an expert, but I think if you're going to take the time to exercise, you should at the very least do a little research to get the maximum benefit.

Through working out, I met and have become close friends with Cal Dietz, who for the past 14 years has been at the University of Minnesota as the strength and conditioning coach for several sports. He has been involved with eight national championship teams and 30 Big Ten title–winning teams including hockey, basketball, baseball, track-and-field, tennis, and golf, to name a handful.

I first met Cal the summer before my freshman year at Hill-Murray, when I participated in his summer conditioning program for hockey. I knew right away there was something special about him, and we seemed to connect early on.

Later that year when my journey in the medical world all began, after many months of setback after setback, surgery after surgery, and the physical toll that went with it, I finally started to come around. It was then that I asked to see Cal. My dad got in touch with him and he came to see me in the hospital. It was the first of many visits. We had many good conversations as the months lingered on, and he was a real inspiration for both me and my family. Just the fact that Cal kept coming was really important to me. He inspired me and gave me lots of words of wisdom. He was a real friend to me, someone to talk to about hockey, conditioning, and life in general. I will always remember what Cal did for me and with me during some very difficult times.

Even when I couldn't walk, I could still work out. My definition of a good workout is one that gets the blood running and the sweat brewing. I like to sweat. When I exercise, I like to set out a specific goal or set of goals and tick them off. Maybe it is to run or walk X number of miles, or to do so many repetitions of a certain exercise, or to do this exercise one day and that one tomorrow. Working out is a challenge, something that anyone can do in any stage of their life—with or without disabilities. I know that for sure because I am living proof that it can be done. I am living proof that getting a desirable workout in is possible. No matter the difficulty of the exercise, I get that familiar feeling when I am done: the feeling of accomplishment and satisfaction. There is nothing else like it.

I am never going to get that sweating, aching, totally-out-of-gas feeling I used to get when a hockey game ended, but I can get close. It is important to me to stay in good shape, to feel good about my body and how I look. I am pretty disciplined when it comes to eating and exercising. Diet is just as important as workouts, and I use good judgment in choosing what I eat—a tall order for a college student with unlimited food at his fingertips! And I always find time in the week to get in my workouts, no matter what else is going on. It is a major part of my life and has helped tremendously in my physical rehab, not to mention my mental state.

Even so, there is no doubt that I do get frustrated, even now. I used to really do fantastic workouts. I would get the very maximum out of my routines. In the beginning after my episode, when I was barely able to do anything, it was pretty defeating. My strength was low, and my muscles did not respond to what I wanted them to do. But I set forth my goals and I worked very hard at achieving them. I wanted desperately to improve and I did, little by little. Even the slightest of improvements has been a big deal for me. When I take something that I cannot do and eventually work hard enough that I can do it again...well, that's huge.

Driving is a good example. Everyone said I could not drive. But I proved them wrong. I did it. I learned how to drive, passed the road test, and defied everybody. Even with my double vision, my dampened depth perception, and everything else that I was experiencing, I did it. The Courage Center, a place that assists those who have suffered short- or long-term disabling injuries by accidents or illnesses assisted me with this, and I had a lot of support from other people too. Yet even with the help and assistance I have received, the bottom line is I have to do it myself. No one else is going to make it happen. I have to count on myself getting it done. It was a tall order, but I have the attitude that when I want to do something, no one is going to be able to discourage me.

There is a time in my life about which I cannot remember much at all. It is a period of a few months right after my injury. I had many crazy dreams during that time, and there are a lot of blanks in my memory bank. The best way I can describe it is to say I was in total despair. Going from a gifted athlete to being rendered virtually helpless is a little more than most people can bear, me included. I had a lot to overcome—a seemingly endless amount. But I did overcome most of it, and today I could not feel better about it. I'm happy, enjoying my life again.

My drive remains the same, but the goals have changed. I used to want to be a hockey player. Now, I'm just not so sure. Today, I'm looking for my true purpose in life. As I have said repeatedly, I do believe my injury happened to me for a reason, and I think it is central to my life's purpose—but I don't know for sure. Maybe it will be to use what happened to me to assist others to get through life-changing events or injuries. I feel confident that I'll know eventually, but for now I know I have to be patient.

Finishing school is a big goal for me too. I wanted to finish high school on time and I did. I never thought for one second that finishing high school would be a goal of mine; it was something I totally took for granted. Of course I would finish on time with all my friends. Why wouldn't I? I had no idea how my life was going to change forever. But it did. No doubt about that. Finishing high school with my peers became a priority, and I did it, despite difficult obstacles. It wasn't easy. I had to relearn everything, take a lot of classes off campus, and do a lot of things I wouldn't have dreamed of.

Going away to college was another of my big goals, and I have done that too. I have some other long-term goals out there, including maybe getting married someday and having a family, but right now college comes first. My education is important to me, and my connection to the hockey team and my friends are big priorities as well.

At this time in my life, I want to do the best I possibly can to be a "normal" person. I work hard at it. Because of the facial problems that have developed, I know I do not look like I used to and I don't look like a normal person. But changing that is a goal I intend to work on. This includes my facial muscles and my eyes. I just want to look like a normal person at some point. Realistically, it may never happen, but that won't be because I haven't given my all to make it happen.

I'm not convinced that my eyes will improve. Maybe they will, but I doubt it. It may be that this is the best they are ever going to be. Maybe they will eventually improve, or maybe medical technology will change, but I doubt it very much. I can accept that and move on. With my face, again, I'm not sure. I have undergone some procedures that have improved things to some extent, but it is a long process. I'm remaining patient.

Sometimes I look at myself in the mirror and ask myself, *Have I done everything I can do to improve my face? Have I done everything I can do to improve my balance, my walking, my reading?* If I have done the best I can possibly do, then I can live with myself, even if the results are not what I hoped for. What I cannot accept is if I haven't given it my best shot.

One of the toughest things I have been working on is getting my balance back in order. This has been difficult. I am pretty good at running, even better than walking. With running, I can spread my base out and the motion comes more naturally. Walking is tougher for me; for whatever reason, putting one foot in front of the other is more of a challenge. I practice it a lot, but I hate doing it. I don't know why the running is better. It seems like it should be the reverse, but it isn't.

Practicing the same repetitive motion day in and day out is really hard for me. It seems so stupid to be doing such basic things, but I know I have to. I understand that these things are a must and that I have to suck it up and get them done if I want to see any kind of improvement.

Writing is a bummer, too. It's really difficult for me to handwrite anything, even a small amount. I'm pretty good on the computer, and that is a good replacement. Reading is another thing that's really difficult for me because of my double vision. My eye muscles don't function the natural way. I'm working on overcoming that, too.

The message here is this: I understand what I can do and what I cannot do. I accept a lot of my abilities that I have come to realize will never be as they used to be. But I am comfortable with that because I know that I am doing all I can do to get better, to improve, and to try to be as normal as possible.

I sometimes put my struggles outside myself, and ask myself how I would respond if someone like me came to me and said, "Look, man, I see double. My face is not what it used to be. I can barely write. I can't read, walk right, talk right, along with a host of other complications and problems. I mean what the hell! I give up." How would I respond to that guy?

To me, it all comes down to your thought process. How do you react to disappointment and misery? How do you react to life-changing experiences? What are you going to do about it?

The way I see it, it's all about effort, effort, effort. You must put effort into something and give it your best, no matter who you are or what you're going through. If you're not going to give it your best, it is not worth trying at all. Either you give 100 percent effort or you give none. Why would anyone facing a life-changing event with an opportunity to improve his overall situation and progress give any less? There is no middle ground. You must give it all to have any chance of improvement. Sure, it is easy to quit, to throw up your hands and give in. I thought about it many times, but I never let it come to pass. I want to be normal, just like everyone else, and I will work the rest of my life to get there.

I relearned so many day-to-day actions. Think about everything you do with your body in a given day. Think about what it takes from your brain and muscles and bones to do anything. Even though we don't consider it oftentimes, those processes are complicated—and I had to learn how to do them all again. I started over.

At the end of the day, when I am 80 years old—if I am fortunate enough to be around that long—I want to and need to look back on my life and say that I never gave up. That comes from me, from no one else but me.

Even considering what I have been through, I think I am for

the most part the same person. I'm still Duke Pieper, but I believe I have expanded my thought process. I think I am a more well-rounded person now. I understand what I have been through and I am proud of it. I survived a 5 percent chance of living, and surmounted so many other obstacles along the way. I feel good about that. It is imbedded in me—the fight, I mean. The fight I have given and continue to give to get better, to survive and to become normal, is what drives me.

One of the toughest things for me is the way some people treat me, look at me, and occasionally respond to some of my disabilities. It's difficult to be judged for who you are on the outside, rather than the inside. But to be perfectly honest, most people are great to me.

I suppose I am the kind of person who appreciates what I do have and does not dwell on what I lost. Call it glass-half-full or whatever you want, but to me it's an important distinction. Some people may look at me and see misfortune, but I feel so fortunate for what I do have. My family loves me. My dog loves me. I have some good friends whom I enjoy being around. I feel I can say that about my life. I really do.

I'm not delusional when it comes to the fact that I will never be the same again. I have problems, I know that. But when you keep in mind the positives in your life and keep the never-give-up attitude on the front burner it will work, I promise. It sure has for me. I may never be the "normal" person I was, but I am going to be very close.

I believe this with every fiber of my heart and soul: Why waste your time on the negative when you can feel good about the positive? And why try to improve what needs improving by giving less than 100 percent of your effort to it? If I don't like how I feel today or I start to dwell on my misfortunes, then I tell myself, *Wake up and do something about it.* There is no other way.

Toughest of Them All

Cal Dietz
University of Minnesota Strength and Conditioning Coach

I HAD A STRENGTH-TRAINING CAMP FOR YOUTH HOCKEY PLAYERS IN THE summer, and that's when I first met Duke Pieper. Duke had been to these kinds of camps in the past, and his dad later told me that initially Duke wasn't all that excited about attending. Later, his dad told me that after the first day, Duke was really fired up about the camp. By the end of the camp, which lasted a few days a week for about six weeks, we had connected some, but then the camp ended and we didn't have any more contact until I heard from his dad some months later.

When Duke first had his medical issues, I did not hear about what happened to him. I know he went through a lot, with the paralysis and all the surgeries. Once Duke was on the road to recovery to the point at least where his family could start communicating with him, I was told he wanted to see me. He actually asked for me to make him stronger again.

Mark didn't remember my name so he contacted Joel Maturi, the athletic director at the University at the time, and found out how to get in touch with me. Mark called me and told me what had happened to Duke. He told me all that had transpired, and I absolutely could not believe it. It bothered me tremendously. As a parent, I was really struck by the pain and agony that Duke's parents must have been going through, watching their son face a horrendous medical condition.

I made arrangements as quickly as I could to see him in the hospital. It really struck me in the heart that he wanted to see me. I know as a coach that we have an impact on the lives of young people. We are in a position to have significant influence and impact but often never know what exactly it is or has been. We lose contact over time and rarely get feedback on whether we helped someone in this way or that way.

With the occasional positive feedback we do get, it is gratifying from time to time to hear that we can make a real difference in young people's lives. I know we do, so that is why all the training and contacts that we have are critical and so important. And I have to say, the results are not just to excel on the ice, the diamond, or wherever, but in life. Hard work, training, and attitude are carryovers to life in general. They provide incredible impact on other parts of one's life in addition to just sports. Duke has been a prime example.

Once I was told of the full severity of what Duke was going through, it really hit me hard. Before I even saw Duke, I was emotionally drained. I recall putting my son to bed that first night after I spoke with Mark and thinking about the impact of something like this on a family. It was very, very hard for me to comprehend something as tragic as this. And he asked to see *me*.

I went to Children's Hospital to see him the following Monday morning. Actually, I had forgotten the name of the hospital he was in and went out to find him. I know that sounds kind of crazy, but it is what happened. I was going to hit every hospital until I found him. By luck, I started with Children's Hospital.

I spent most of the morning talking with the family and communicating with Duke as much as I could. From that time on, I went to see him about twice a week. His spirits raised some when I showed up, so I was really glad about that. I wanted no recognition for any of this and still do not want any. I was just glad we had connected and that I was able to provide some type of assistance for him and what he was going through.

Over time he got better, and we would have conversations about never quitting, always moving ahead. We talked about all kinds of things and the importance of maintaining a positive attitude and moving in a forward direction. We never did actual workouts together; it was mostly just spending time together talking and enjoying each other's company. I felt from just the short time we had at my training camp that he had the tools to someday become an elite hockey player. I saw that in him. So to see him in the "then" and "now" was hard for me to comprehend.

I can remember going with his parents once while we helped him walk around the block. That was a tough day, and it wasn't about me, it was about him—and I had to keep reminding myself of that fact. I did whatever I could to keep him motivated, keep his spirits up, and keep him moving in the right direction.

It has been an amazing experience for me to be involved with Duke. For what happened to him and the way he keeps going, not giving up, he has to be one of the toughest individuals I have ever come in contact with in my life. I have trained great athletes, world champions, and I don't know many people, if any, who could have suffered what he has suffered and still have the attitude he has.

I'm sure there have been times when he has questioned God, questioned his parents and life in general, but the mere fact that he has kept his head up and kept going says a lot. I deal with tough human beings in my job every day, from wrestlers to hockey players, and I have seen that sometimes when something catastrophic happens to them they shut down, they never make it back. In Duke's case, he suffered a life-changing experience and has proven how you can control one thing for sure, and that is your outlook on life. Your attitude will guide you along the way.

Duke is different. He is special. He controls his life through his attitude. He likely was given great guidance from his parents and through his participation in sports. He has the resolve to move ahead. It is easy to tell from the contact I had with the family that Duke and his sister have been the focal point of Mark and Liz Pieper. They have provided the nucleus to get him through this, combined with his great attitude and resourcefulness.

I think that, for sure, every person should hear this story, *his* story. Especially young people—I think they need to hear something like this. I think it is an example of how much one needs to appreciate what they have because they can lose it so quickly—and if they do suffer some of life's perils, how to move on, move ahead. Duke has raised the bar in that regard.

Duke had a great gift to play hockey and he lost it, but it has not held him back. Anyone, at any time, can lose what he has. It may be an illness, a car accident, anything. We all have to be grateful for what we have in life because in an instant it can be taken from us.

We often look at sports as the greatest of things, but they are not. It is more important to be a great parent, a great friend, a great family member, a great person. To never disregard this and never give up when you have setbacks in life is the key. And Duke exemplifies this in spades, over and over. He is an amazing individual and I am proud to know him and be a part of his life.

CHAPTER 10

A Lot of Doubts (Not Mine)

After being admitted to the hospital, things took a turn for the worse. My condition was bad enough that most of the people around me did not think I was going to live. I was only told later about my 5 percent chance of survival. Those are not very good odds, so I suppose it's understandable that they didn't tell me from the start.

I was in pretty bad shape, but here I am. I made it. Mind over matter. Because of everything that had occurred, there were a lot of doubts about my future. My doctors and my family did not know what I was going to be able to do. How was I going to move forward? How was I going to be able to function? Would I be able to live a normal life again? These were essential questions, but the answers were far from certain. Doubt clouded everything.

If I was on the outside looking in, I suppose I would have the same reservations. *Look at him. He is never going to be able to walk again. He will never run, read, or write. I mean, the kid cannot even breathe on his own! His vision is shot. Playing hockey again? Out of the question. He is never going to be able to go to school again.* I understand why people thought such things; I would likely have agreed with them if I had been looking in at myself objectively. I was a mess.

I had very little I could do at the time. I had virtually no muscle at all. I had nystagmus in my eyes, which is a form of involuntary eye movement; I saw two of everything. My disabilities were countless. I had become helpless. The prospects of me being able to live much of a normal life looked pretty dim.

In the very beginning, I could not function at all. Slowly but surely, I learned to eat, walk, breathe, and swallow again. Still, as I improved, things like driving were so incredibly far away that they seemed to fall into the category of the impossible. But not to me; I never had a doubt that I would drive again. I truly knew that if I was going to have any kind of life again, I would have to be able to drive and get myself from place to place. Without the ability to drive a vehicle I would be totally dependent upon someone else getting me to where I wanted to go.

I had no doubt in my mind that I would be able to drive, despite what anyone else thought. I knew in the very depths of my soul that I would try and try and try again until I could do it. My mom and dad helped me a lot by giving me a great deal of their time. I had a lot of help, and a lot of love and support. When I was ready, I took the driving test at a Department of Motor Vehicles office—and I passed with flying colors, to my tremendous satisfaction. I showed those people with doubts that I could do it. Not to brag, but the fact is that there are some able-bodied people who cannot pass the first time, second time, and in some cases after many attempts. To say I was proud of my achievement would be an understatement.

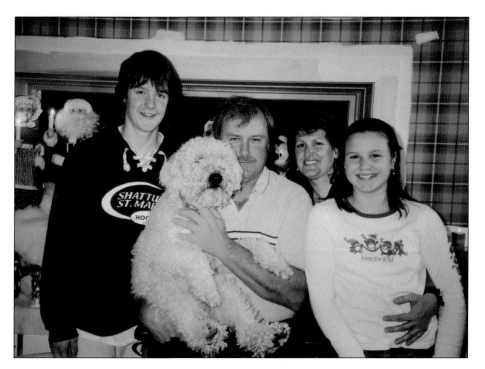

With my wonderful family: Christmas 2011.

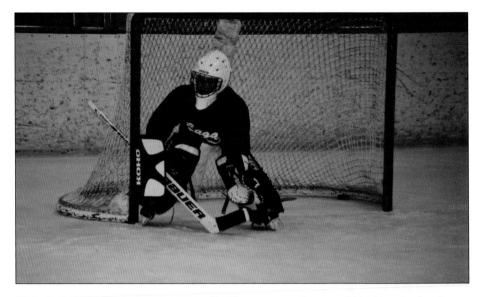

I began my hockey career as a goalie. You can see how well that worked out (check out the puck in the corner of the net).

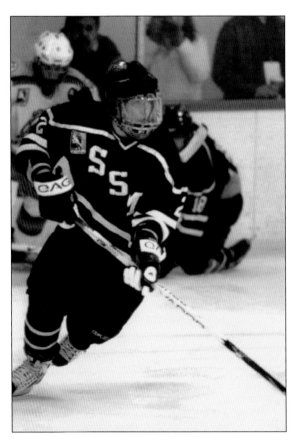

By the time I was playing at Shattuck–St. Mary's, I was firing on all cylinders.

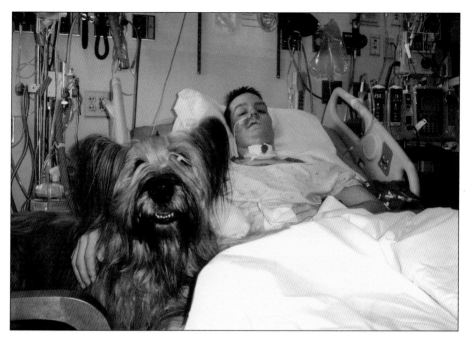

Pepsi was a frequent hospital visitor.

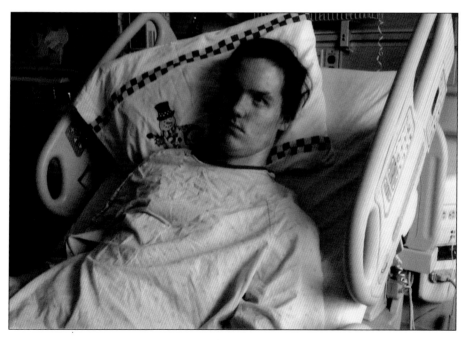

All that time in the hospital took its toll. I was ready to go home.

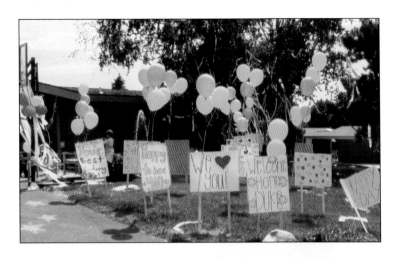

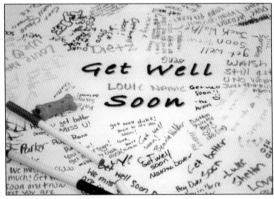

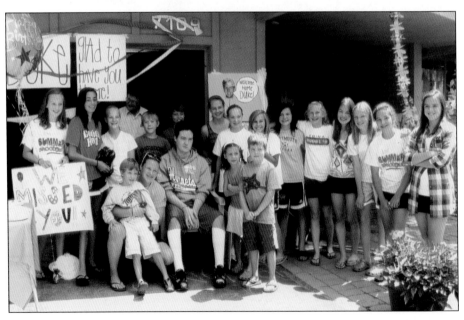

My homecoming was extremely special.

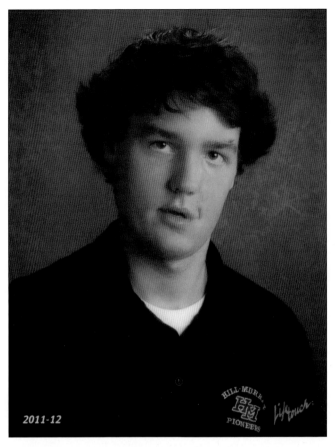

Returning to Hill-Murray and graduating with my class was a huge priority.

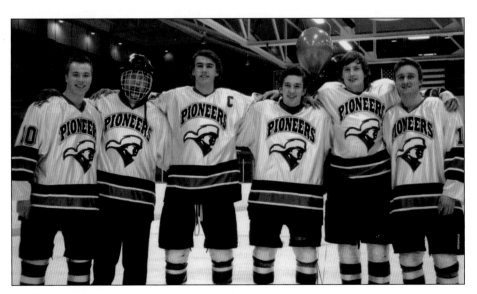

On the ice with my Hill-Murray teammates.

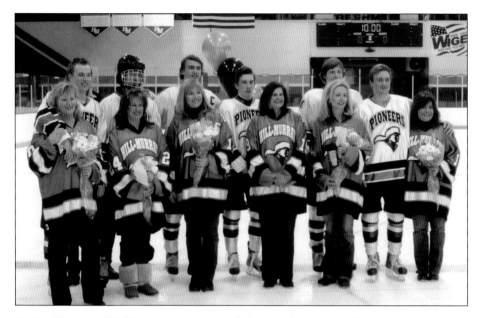

Senior Night at Hill-Murray was so special. A celebration of all the hard work the senior hockey players put in, it was especially poignant for me.

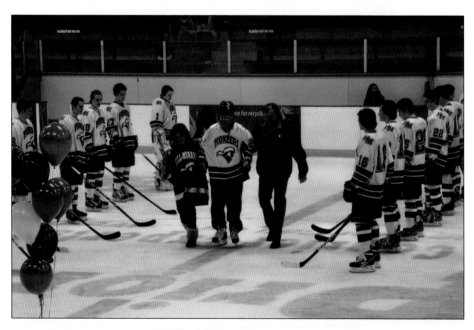

I was particularly grateful to share that night with my parents and thank them for all their sacrifices.

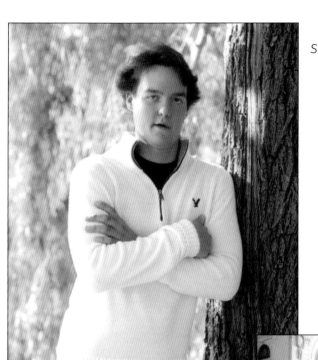

Senior portrait.

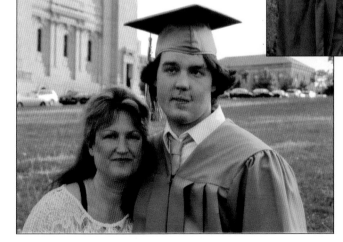

Graduation at Hill-Murray. I did it!

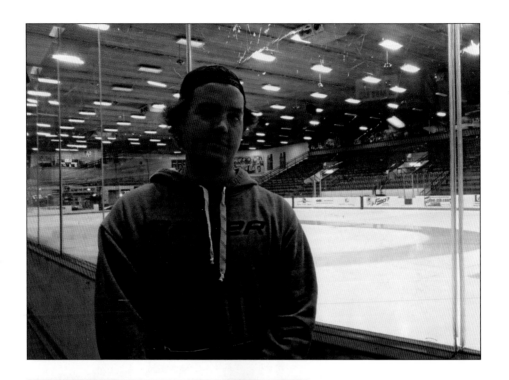

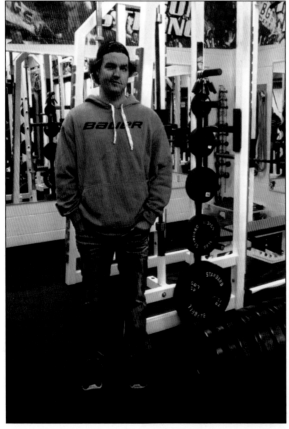

Thrilled to be on my own at Bowling Green State University. Here I am at some of my frequent on-campus haunts: the arena and the weight room.

A lot of people also doubted whether or not I would ever be able to go to a regular school again. High school seemed to them unlikely, and college impossible. When I was in the hospital on the verge of dying, I don't think there were very many people who would have thought in a million years that I would go to college. And here I am today, going to college out of state, at Bowling Green in Ohio, all by myself. I didn't know a soul when I enrolled at Bowling Green, and I have managed to succeed there on my own. It makes me proud that I have not only defied but absolutely shattered people's doubts about me.

I often wonder what is in store for me in the future. I'm excited to look ahead, excited about the possibilities, whatever they may be. All I know for sure is that I'll carry my positive attitude and go after my goals, even under the most difficult of circumstances. In my situation, I think many people would have given up or at least not put in the effort. That's not me, and it never will be. But I'm not trying to say I am anything special. I just mean that no matter what roadblock is in my way, I have always been able to find a way to get through it. And I've encountered some pretty big, pretty unexpected roadblocks along the way.

I think it comes from being a hockey player, at least to some extent. When my team was down by five goals in a game, I never gave up. I have always been that way. The competitive fire in me is never extinguished. I recall a time when I was playing a game and it was late in the third period and our team was behind by three goals. It looked like it was over for sure, but our team never gave up and we rallied and wound up winning the game. It was a good lesson for the whole team. Never fall to the level of "It's over."

I have always held on to this mentality. I think some of that comes from my dad and seeing how hard he works, and seeing my mom and how she is so good at taking care of everything. The success I have had and the progress I have made since my brain injury have built the foundation for my beliefs that never giving up can yield some extraordinary results.

One minute I was a normal kid doing anything I wanted to do, and the next minute every single thing in my life had changed. I recall being in the hospital and going down the hallway with my walker, two people on each side of me, a belt on my waist to hold me up, thinking, *Are you kidding me? One minute I am racing across the blue line with the puck and the next minute this?*

It was the beginning, though some might have referred to it as the end. But because of all that I have been brought up with and learned, it was not going to be that way for me. My life was not over. It was the beginning. And I got through it. I'm right here. I wrote this book, and now I'm telling others about my story. Like I have said so many times before, I believe that anything you want to accomplish in life is right there for the taking—and I am taking it with a hop, skip, and a jump.

I have come to understand that nothing comes easy. No matter what you are able to accomplish, no matter how many barriers you overcome, there is still plenty of pain and disappointment along the way. That is a given and a part of what has to be overcome in the process.

I recall some time ago being invited to a party that included many of my friends, former teammates, and current hockey players. Several were playing college hockey and I had played with a number of them at one time or another. And there were others there, too, including a guy who was playing in the NHL for the Chicago Blackhawks. It was a fun night, it really was, but after the night was over, everything kind of hit me—and hit me hard.

Here were all these guys I knew, all healthy and living their dream—my dream. Many were on college teams, doing well, and hoping that maybe they could play professionally someday. And there was the guy living his dream, playing in the NHL. I was in the same room with a guy who played for the Blackhawks—and they won the Stanley Cup championship. That was *my* dream— and he was my age and I had played against him at one time. It was hard not to feel devastated.

Seeing all these guys, all the fun they were having, all the success they were having...it hit me hard. And then there was me. I wasn't the same person. I didn't look the same, talk the same, and had a list of problems too long to count. It wasn't fair. It sucked. I hated it. I felt sorry for myself, big-time. But that feeling didn't last long. I wouldn't let it. It was not me and was not going to be me.

I have never asked myself how to get through the moments like that; I suppose the best way to say it and get through it is to simply accept it. Like I said before, there is a choice you have to make here. You can feel sorry for yourself and let that consume you and take over your life, or you can accept it and move ahead. Feeling sorry for myself will not change a single thing. That realization came to me early on, and it has made all the difference.

So buckle up. Get over it. Move on. There may never be a time when you totally accept this kind of defeat, but if you can stay positive for the most part, I believe you are on the right track. It's not easy, but there are strategies that work for me to keep me going. After a night like that, when reality really hits me, I have to find a way to get through it. Usually what works best for me is to go out and do something I enjoy doing. I find something that keeps my mind on the right track and gets me feeling good again. Finding that something positive is my medicine. It dampens the hurt and brings me back to reality so that I can move on.

Working out tends to relieve a lot of my stress. That has always been something that can get me in the right frame of mind. Any kind of physical activity—running, lifting weights, even walking—clears my mind, and in actuality it does much more than that. It just gives me a good feeling all over.

When I wake up in the morning I try to start the day with a good attitude. And I can honestly say that most days I do just that. I try to always understand that I have to accept what has happened to me, as difficult as it is sometimes, and move forward. *Today is going to be a good day. I'm going to feel good today*, I tell myself. It works well for me.

There are so many things that keep me positive, but physical conditioning is first and foremost. Of course, there are days that I can't work out for one reason or another. When that becomes the case, then I know I have to find other ways to keep my mind right. I try to find other things to do or think about, even if it's just little things. So think of something positive. Evaluate the kind of state you are in. Ask yourself, *Do I like how I feel today?* If the answer is no, then do something about it.

Another method that works for me is to recall what I have been through over the months and years. I look to the past and compare that to where I am in the present. It's miles apart, being on the edge of death to where I am now.

As I venture back, I remember wondering what it would feel like to die. I asked my dad about it: "What is it like to die?" I needed two people to hold me up just so I could take a few steps. I had lost everything in my life physically. I could not do a single thing on my own. So eating, swallowing, breathing on my own, driving, that became my ultimate goal—until I achieved it, and then set a new goal for myself.

Most athletes enjoy the feeling of winning the big game. I don't know how to put it into words that do it justice, but there is a special feeling you get when you win the big one. Those who have played sports know what I mean. It is something inside you that is a really special feeling. I don't see myself ever getting that feeling again playing sports; that part of my life is over for me. So I have to find it other places—and I have.

Succeeding academically is a good start. A 3.0 grade-point average is not bad. Doing well doesn't give me that championship-game euphoria, but it's good. I think in my situation, I have to continue to let my mind take me to the right places. Going away to school by myself and doing well is absolutely a good feeling. It may not be the overwhelming feeling of scoring the game-winning goal, but in the grand scope of things, taking into account what I have been through, I think it is much, much bigger.

Music is another great outlet for me. Even on some of my worst days, it makes me feel good. My hearing is perfect, and I am thankful for that. My friends are there for me, too, and I have made a lot of new friends. They are different from the type of people who were in my life. Which is not to say I have rejected the people in my life beforehand, it's just that I have broadened my horizons when it comes to people. I used to only hang with the athletes, the hockey guys. I still do, but not all the time. I have had the opportunity to meet people with other interests, and that has been good for me. I'm not a hockey player anymore and I have accepted that. I never thought that would be a positive thing, but it is. I've become involved in so many other things as a result. Before, my friends were part of a pretty narrow group, so I know overall I have grown. I think being more inclusive is all good. I believe I am a better person, a wiser person, and I like myself better than before. I really do.

I enjoy being around people. I admire the "nice guy," and I want to be that kind of person. I want to be the caring person, the compassionate person. I work at it, and hope I am seen that way by those who know me. I strive to develop the good qualities in myself. I know I screw up and let myself down from time to time, but I do my very best to be mindful of the person I want to be.

I was in a box before, living a dream. It was not all good—not bad, nor ideal either. Some of the things I now see as important in life weren't even on my radar then. I want to learn, have some intelligence, be nice to people, care about people, and be looked upon as a really nice person. Before, I never thought about any of those things. Now this is important to me.

As a result of what happened to me, there are some very important things in life that have jumped to my front burner. I feel good about rearranging my perspective. There have been some good things that have come about as a result of my life-changing experience, and broadening my horizons is one of the big ones.

What I am about to say might sound unnatural or maybe even ridiculous, but I am going to say it anyway. Despite everything, in so many ways I am happy about what happened to me. Happy because it changed me in many ways for the better. It sounds crazy, but it made me realize a lot about my life. It made me look back at what kind of person I was before and see myself with clear eyes. There were things I didn't like about myself. To put it bluntly, I was a jerk. No one likes to be self-critical, but I was.

I was so caught up in hockey, with all my success, that some of the really important things in life had passed me by. Paying the price of losing my dream was devastating, but so many good things have come from it. More important things now have taken over my attention. I am getting a good education and am engaged in the process of learning. I am forging new relationships with a variety of people.

This new lease on life is incredible, and I'm extremely grateful for it. Still, if I were to say that every single day is now a bed of roses because I have accepted my new life and my worldview, I would not be telling the truth. It is still hard. I struggle but try my best to keep everything I possibly can in a positive light. When I have those moments, they don't last long. I won't let them.

Someone once asked me how I could see what happened to me as a good thing. The person, frankly, was puzzled by my positive outlook. I said it's because I know I am a better person now. This has opened up my eyes to so many different things, and I feel really good about living in the world I now am a part of, which is so different from the past.

When I look in the mirror, for the most part I feel pretty good. Do I like myself? Most of the time. That can be a little harder. When I was finally released from the hospital, I have to admit I was a very messed-up individual. I had to find a way to accept that person. He wasn't me. He wasn't the same. Everything about him was different, from physical appearance to abilities. I have come to accept the fact that I am me, even if a slightly different version.

My heart is the same. I think it is a good heart—at least I try hard to have a good heart, to do the right thing, to be honest and treat others well. These are important values for me now, values I should have had before but didn't put as much emphasis on. I guess they were always there within me; it just took something big to get them out. I'm glad they're at the forefront now.

It was tough but I finally told myself, *Look, this is what I have to deal with now. This is what I have to work with. What are my choices?* Even while I was still a hospital patient, I made an important choice. I had the opportunity to be prescribed some medication that would assist me in coping emotionally. Not one time did I take any of that medication. Not once. I had a pretty good idea of what lay ahead of me, and it seemed overwhelming. But I was determined to deal with it myself, not with the help of some drugs. I am not saying that everyone facing similar circumstances should follow that same path, but I did what I thought was the best thing for me.

Since my hospital release, there have been so many obstacles to overcome, and I have worked hard to beat most of the odds stacked against me. I will never give up on my goals. I will never let doubts prevent me from going for what I am able to accomplish in my life.

I still want the good things in life; I haven't given up on them. I know I will have to work a little harder to get certain things, but giving up, giving in, having doubts? Not a chance. Not for one moment will I let that stand in my way. *Doubt* is not a word in my vocabulary.

Keep Telling the Story

Larry Hendrickson
Minnesota High School Hockey Coaches Hall of Fame Member
and Founder of the Hendrickson Foundation

LET ME BEGIN BY SAYING THIS ABOUT MY FRIEND DUKE PIEPER. OF ALL THE people I have met in my life, his character, his depth, is as high as any one person I have ever met. Furthermore, he has had an incredible impact on my life. I don't think I would be doing some of the things I am doing today if it had not been for people like Duke who have influenced me the way they have. And I can honestly say I am specifically referencing Duke when I say this. He has such high values and is an outstanding human being.

He gets it. Duke Pieper gets it. What I have just said are some pretty strong comments to make about anyone, but I can tell you that Duke has earned every one of those words. We are all human beings, meaning we all have strengths and we all have weaknesses.

Most people I know are 90 percent good and have maybe 10 percent of things that they have to work on. We are mostly self-centered to some degree, and that's okay, because some of that is a good thing. In some ways we have to be to meet our various duties and responsibilities. But there is a time when most human beings think, *What is in this for me? What do I get out of this?* Yet with Duke—and it pops up constantly when I am with him—his main focus is always, *How does this, whatever it might be, affect others? How does this affect someone else?* He is not like many people who think of themselves first—not this young man.

Duke is very selfless. He has this great gift to constantly think about others. He is basically a good, giving, caring, and selfless person. I don't know how saints are picked—trust me, I am about the last guy to be doing that kind of endeavor—but it is my guess that some of the qualities of those who are picked are centered in Duke as well.

He not only has these tremendous attributes when it comes to others, but he also has made his own personal connection with God. God is a strong force in his life, an important reality for him. It is not a "maybe, I'm not sure" kind of thing but an everyday thought. Those kinds of things about Duke Pieper have an impact on me personally. He makes a difference in my life by my knowing him, by him being the kind of person he is, and by the very fact that he is instrumental in bringing a positive spirit to my life. He has a strong faith, and it rubs off. It certainly has rubbed off on me.

For him to be able to handle what he has gone through and to be able to keep such a wonderful attitude is a mystery to me. I cannot understand what drives him to be the special person he is. My guess is that his mom and dad have had a huge impact on him being the way he is. I don't know his mom very well, other than knowing she is a good person, a good mom. I know his dad, Mark, much better and know he is a giving, loving person, and I know they both have had great influence on Duke.

However, for Duke to be the kind of person he is, I think it goes much deeper than that. I think somehow he has gotten himself closely connected to his God. That's what I think. Do I know? No, I don't know, but I do know how important his God is to him. I mean, that's where his power and strength to move ahead comes from. I believe that. I really do, but this in reality is deeper than I want to go. When I see this and believe this about him, it has an impact on me and I grow from that. I learn from him. I actually ask myself, *How can I be more*

Duke-like? I want to have the abilities that Duke has to make a difference in others' lives.

I made that comment to someone once about being more Duke-like. The person asked me how old I was and I replied that I was 71. The person then responded back (in an inquisitive but positive manner) by asking, "How is it that a young man 20 years old can have such an impact on someone at the age of 71?" I answered the question by saying that I love youth, first of all. I really do. Young people inspire me and I love to be around them. I actually believe I get along better with young people than I do with older people, mostly because they all have so many dreams and hopes. They are not afraid of change. Life is full of change and it is tougher for older people, those my age, to accept change. We get set in our ways. I recall growing up, and my parents thought the world was coming to an end with the "hippie era" and all those protests against the government. I'm kind of like that, you know, getting nervous about new things and changes. Anyway, Duke has that incredible spirit of the young person. He delivers an impact to others, to me. There have been a lot of young people that have provided a huge impact for me like Duke. He is off the charts in that regard, a leader.

I work with disabled athletes who have lost limbs while in military war zones, who play sled hockey, having to utilize a sled they rest on. They tell me, like Duke does, "Don't tell me what I have lost but tell me what I can do, what I have." They believe it is their job to influence others. Duke represents that same value system. He has an insight that is so positive, so giving, so caring that it has an impact on everyone who comes in contact with him. I enjoy watching him. I enjoy the influence he has on others while taking in his influence myself as well. It is absolutely amazing to me to watch those he has affected in so many different ways.

Duke often talks about believing that what happened to him was supposed to happen. "There was a reason for this," he says. If this is true, and I don't know that it is, then I believe he has faithfully turned to God to deal with it. It certainly could be true, but the fact is I don't know how God works in these situations. Now, I *can* say I know how Duke works. I know that whatever comes his way, he is going to deal with it in the most positive way possible.

For example, some time back not too long after we first met, I was at a Minnesota Wild game with Duke and his dad. It was a very tough time for all concerned. Duke's medical problems had really come to the forefront, and some really difficult decisions had to be made to treat his ailment. The decisions were life-threatening. As close as I was to Duke back then, I cannot imagine what he and his parents were going through. It was a tough spot to be in, and it was very hard on the family at the time. During the intermission between periods at the game, Duke had left the seats to go and get some food. Mark began telling me about the situation they were facing. It became quite emotional, and Mark started crying as he was telling me about it. Soon Duke returned to the seats and noticed his dad was talking to me with tears in his eyes. Duke instantly assessed what was happening and immediately said to Mark, "Dad, Dad, knock it off. I told you before, the worst scenario is that I will make it to heaven before you." And then we got back to the game and we had a fun time the rest of the night. Duke intervened and made it better for both of us. He knew what he had to do and he responded perfectly.

I was very fortunate to meet Duke. I met him through my son, Darby, who is now assistant coach with the Minnesota Wild. He had finished his career playing professionally and was working for Fox Sports North. It was "Hockey Night in Minnesota," and as a part of the day, Duke had been selected to drop the puck in the pregame ceremony.

Former St. Paul Johnson High School legendary coach Lou Cotroneo was being honored before the game, and then Duke was to drop the ceremonial puck. Darby and Duke had not met previously, but something affected Darby about their meeting. He recognized right away what a tremendously special person Duke was. He came to me and said, "Dad, you have got to meet this kid." We hit it off immediately, and I saw the same thing that my son had seen. What a special kid! We really bonded and started going to some Wild games together. I became close to Mark Pieper, and we all had a really fun time together. It was a true pleasure. We went to games and out to eat after and had some wonderful times. I spent a lot of time with Duke and his dad. Often Darby would join us, too, and that really was a great time. Duke just enjoys life.

I have so appreciated our connection, and it brought me to one of the most humbling experiences of my life. Duke asked me if I would come on the ice at the Hill-Murray Senior Night for the varsity hockey players. This was a couple years after we first met. The traditional night involved the senior players being introduced before the final home game, and they skated on the ice and greeted their parents. Duke, an honorary team captain, asked me to be there with his parents. I cannot begin to explain what that meant to me.

I chose not to go on the ice with his mom and dad, as I felt it was a special time for them, so I waited nearby in the players' box. Duke was still in very tough physical condition and had to be assisted by players and then his parents as he came on the ice with the rest of his senior team. Still, he took the time to come over and give me a loving hug. It gives me chills to recall that special night with this incredible young man. For me to be a part of that evening was so incredibly meaningful. It is also extremely humbling to me that Duke picked me as one of the people to have an opportunity to be a part of his book. That also has really meant a great deal to me. I feel honestly I don't deserve this. I am deeply honored to be a part of something that has become so important to him.

Duke has the ability to let people know that he cares about them. It seems like he always grabs on to the opportunity to let people know how he feels about them and he does it in such a positive manner.

I ran the Select 15 Hockey Camp for young players and I had Duke come to the camp and speak. He was outstanding. What I recall is that he told the kids how important it is to be thankful for the gifts you have been given in life. And further, to be thankful to the people who have contributed to those gifts. It was amazing because, as I mentioned before, I have been around a lot of people who have lost arms and legs and now play sled hockey. They are so thankful for what they have and do not dwell on what they lost. Duke does such a terrific job of conveying that message to others: "Reach your potential. Be a positive influence in others' lives." It is such a great message.

When I am around people like I mentioned and people like Duke, I am the happiest I have ever been in my life. Their philosophy means so much to me and to others who hear it. It actually might make a good guy out of me someday.

I think it is really important for people to recognize in life that absolutely nothing is guaranteed. All that you have can be taken away in a flash, an instant. Obviously people can make bad decisions that lead to tragedy, but even if you do everything the right way, tragedy can still come about. It's just the way the world works. I see that time and time again with injuries, sickness, and other life-changing experiences.

Duke Pieper has many attributes, but being respectful of others may in fact top the list. He is aware of what is going on around him, knows the difficulty that some people have in dealing with what he has gone through, and tries to make it easy for people. He is the one with the problems, and yet is so respectful of others that he worries about making people uncomfortable around him. That very attribute speaks to his character and his heart.

Before we met, I had heard very little about Duke. I guess I knew of him somewhat from other people. As I recall, the only thing I did know was he was supposedly this great athlete at Shattuck–St. Mary's, an even better student, and an even better person. I knew the Hill-Murray hockey coach well—that would be Bill Lechner, whom I have as much respect for as any coach in hockey today. I remember asking him once about Duke. I asked him, "What is this Duke Pieper like as a player?" The answer from Bill was all superlatives. He absolutely raved about his abilities as a freshman player, maybe one of the best to ever come into the school as a ninth-grader, he said. I was told of his athletic brilliance, his prominence, and then, *boom*, the curve ball came.

I am so glad Duke is doing this book. His story has to be told. I think it is so important that others hear what he has gone though and what he has to say. I think all of us as human beings need to come in contact with people and ideas that are bigger than we are. It is important for our human race. We need to hear these kinds of inspirational stories to better understand ourselves, to understand what we have and what we need to be thankful for in our lives. Duke had everything going for him and lost it all. And look at him: he is more grateful, more thankful than bunches of us all put together.

We can look at life and see people who take everything they can get from everyone or anyone. Those people have no pride, no honesty, no integrity. And then we have saints on the other side. But most of us fall in the middle. And we need to hear heartfelt stories because it is a reminder of what we have and have failed to appreciate. People need to hear Duke's story. His story makes all of us stronger people. We can learn from what he has to tell us.

I never worry about what Duke might say. He speaks from the heart. I believe his message is a strong, spiritual one, and whatever is supposed to happen with his message through his book will happen. Jesus said, "Don't worry about the results. Keep telling the story." I believe this is appropriate here. Keep telling the story. Keep moving on. Changing even one person's life is significant.

When we have a curve ball in our lives—and most of us will have one to some degree while we are on earth—we need to hear about the strength of people like Duke and understand how he has fought the battle by never giving in, never giving up. He has been an unbelievable inspiration to so many and has undoubtedly proven his strength and passion for life.

CHAPTER 11

Some Good Thoughts

I have learned a few things over the past months and years since my world initially collapsed. I guess that is a pretty good way to say it—*collapsed*, I mean. But look how far I have come.

Right off the top of my head, I have learned firsthand that when you put a little bit of effort into something, good things can happen. The results can be big with significant effort. All the effort I have put into recovering from my disabilities has proven how far I have come toward my goal of being normal again someday. I have definitely noticed the improvement.

Even with significantly impaired eyesight, I have learned how to safely drive a car. Learning to walk again was tough, but I always knew deep down I was going to overcome that huge challenge; I just knew I would. But driving? That seemed, at one point, so far off. I could not imagine even thinking about it, let alone doing it. Of course, that changed.

I'm not sure if I can ever count on my eyes to fully recover, but

I have noticed improvement when I do certain kinds of exercises. For example, with practice, I am able to distinguish which image I see and which eye is the proper one to focus on. This did not come naturally to me. I had to work at it. It helped me to get the images to become more distinct and made everything much more clear for me. I got assistance from someone who worked with people who have eye problems. It was not an eye doctor or a specialist but rather a rehab person. He worked with me to utilize different muscles in the eyes to improve my vision and perspective. I don't know all the technological terms or methods he employed, but I learned how to compensate.

The simple things in life, things that people do every single day of their lives, things that I used to do every day of my life, have created troubles for me. Going up and down the stairs at home was a big task at first. When I first got out of the hospital, it was a huge obstacle to overcome. Railings were the thing that saved me. In the beginning when I left the hospital, stairs without railings were troubling to say the least; a better word is *frightening*. When I re-enrolled at Hill-Murray, the stairs were daunting, but I still made it through. Of course, it wasn't just managing to get myself up or down, it was managing to get up and down while also carrying a load of heavy school books. Sometimes, I wonder how I ever navigated it. These days, I am pretty good at climbing and descending stairs, but I am still careful. I can't describe what a great feeling it is. I can still remember so vividly how terrifying it was at first.

I have come to understand that all of the frustrations and difficulties I have faced over the years are a part of the process. You have no choice but to face what life hands you head-on. You have to work through it. If you stumble once, twice, three times, or four times, you get back up and you try again. There are no other options to consider. You face it again and again and again. It's simply the way it is.

Sure, giving up is always an option—it's just not an acceptable one. I let surrendering cross my mind early on, but only for a brief moment. And then everything I have ever believed in my life kicked in; surrender was no longer an option for me.

There is no question that if I rated my satisfaction in how my life is going, I would not be at the top of my personal scale. But I know that someday I will look back on all this and see that I gave life everything I had. I never gave up. I was the best version of myself I could be. And I will be profoundly proud of where I come from. That will be a very important moment in my life.

I don't spend a lot of time focusing on any of the particular physical actions I do differently from others—such as walking, eating, seeing, and going up and down the stairs, just to name a few. Instead, it is much more important to focus on my inner strength and how I use that strength to overcome life's perils. I believe that this strength is ingrained in me, and I use it to summon my best efforts in getting as close to normal as possible. I want to be the guy out there who can do everything.

Sometimes I fall short. It's a battle I fight when things don't go so well, when they don't go as planned. I think back on how angry I was in the beginning.

My relationship with God has had its rough times. We were at odds for a period of time. I guess I could comfortably say that we were not the best of friends. But my religious faith rose up and took over, and we are back in good graces again. At the time, I felt as if I had to have someone to blame for what happened to me; God happened to be at whom I pointed my finger. I know now that God is with me, not against me.

The process of recovery is long and winding and there are so many parts to it. One of those parts has been the development of my faith and relationship with God. It has made me so strong in my daily battle to become a person who can do things on his own. He has been there for me and helped me tremendously. He inspired me to keep putting one foot in front of the other each day. He kept my drive and my effort focused and moved me forward.

I was angry with God at the beginning, but as time went on I changed my thinking. I feel very strongly that there is a reason for what has happened to me. I have a purpose in life relative to the moment I came off the ice before my first high school hockey game with Hill-Murray. I will answer that call, wherever it takes me. Until I know just what that is, I will keep striving for my goals and being the best person I can be.

My religion and my belief in God have helped me through some of my most difficult times. In Philippians 1:6, God makes a promise that what he starts in our lives he will finish. He doesn't forget and he doesn't give up. He simply will never start what he cannot finish. God has put hope in our hearts that if things don't work out and do not happen, then He will say it is not over and that He has the final say to begin again.

Even to this day, I still have rough nights when I think of the past, and the pain is sometimes unbearable. But I think my way through it and know that God's arms rest on my shoulders and that I am going to be okay. I will get through it and in the end I will be better for it.

I don't know exactly what is in store for me; no one ever really does. But what I do know is that I am not alone. I have my family. I have my friends. I have God at my side, seeing me through. And it is this that is comforting for me as I move ahead.

This has been a literal godsend for me: a hope and a prayer that keeps me going with the belief that I will go on—and I will go on with a mission at hand. I feel that I was truly saved from dying more than once, and I can say that I truly was saved like Christ was when he rose from the dead into heaven. I have a pretty good idea what is in store for me. I believe there is a plan, and that I will embark on that plan and be a light and a guide for others. I truly believe I have been given a gift to pass on to others who so desperately need a guide to face life's challenges.

My ultimate goal was once to play on a hockey team that wins the Stanley Cup. There is a part of me that has never given up on that hope, and for the most part I think it's okay to think about that from time to time. Then there is another part of me that is reality-driven, telling me it is not going to happen. Even so, I know almost anything is possible. I can certainly look back at the early stages of my injury and recognize that no one ever believed I would be where I am today.

I mean, I had a 5 percent chance of living! My family was making funeral arrangements for me! Then later, in recovery, I couldn't walk, talk, swallow, or even breathe. I mean, come on here—finish high school and go to college away from home and across the country? No way! But here I am. So there is no doubt miracles can happen. Playing on a championship hockey team… well, you just never know.

I look at life differently now. I look at others who are facing difficulties and I can relate to what they are going through. I understand the pain and the perils they face in life every single day. Beforehand, I never gave other people's troubles much of a thought. Now I can have empathy for them.

I have come to understand that a life-changing episode or experience can alter one's dreams and change them forever. I understand the challenges one can face ahead and the rough times some people will face. Does this make me a better person? I guess I'm not really sure about that. But what I do know is that I care more about others, and I think about things more than I used to.

I'm all for helping out people who need it. Sometimes it can be the little things. I look for those moments, those opportunities. Doing for others makes me feel good, and I guess it makes me a better person.

I know that as I meet my future, I will employ these changes in myself to hopefully become an inspiration for others. I can do this because, humbly speaking, there is no question that I have become an inspiration for myself. To use (what else?) a hockey metaphor, I am in the big game and the team is winning. We were behind early but have been coming on strong, and with the help and grace of God, the light burns brighter as the game gets into the second period. I know there is a long way to go, and my attitude and inspiration will endure with my unrelenting faith. And in the end, victory will be achieved and I will cherish the moment.

Sometimes I get frustrated when I think about the things I used to be able to do and can't anymore. Most of the time the things I cannot do physically cause me the most grief. I get so mad. I'll admit I have developed somewhat of a temper, and I don't like that about myself. I have definitely noticed I get much more edgy than I used to before my problems began. Frustration seems to set in with a vengeance, and I get irritated faster than I did when I was functioning normally. I guess it is good to realize it, and have to keep working to better myself in that area. I know there is no excuse for that behavior, and that nothing good can come from it.

I try hard not to show my frustration, and sometimes that can become a problem because I tend to keep things bottled up inside. Unless you are in my world, walking a mile in my shoes, it's impossible to know how I feel. I really do understand how difficult it is for anyone to relate to how I'm feeling.

I can recall a time after I had recovered considerably when I went to a game. I was not able to step up on the bleachers. It really frustrated me and I got very angry. I mean, step up on the bleachers! Before I never gave it a thought. But then I had to step back and think, *Well, I guess I can wait for this bleacher thing because there was a time when I couldn't walk.*

Sometimes I have to take a hard look at where I was before all this happened and where I am at the present point. Say there is a scale of normalcy, rated 1 through 10, 10 being the most normal. Where I was before my injury was the max, a strong 10. I went 10 to 1 virtually overnight. But since then, I've been moving gradually up the scale. It is one step at a time, one little increment at a time, but it is slow but sure progress. As I write this part of the book, I think I'm at about a 5 on the scale. I say this because in my way of counting, I am a long way from a 10 and an equally long way from that 1, which is equivalent to rock bottom. As long as my number is increasing, I'm happy. Progress. Progress. Progress.

Before all this started, I was a 10 without even thinking about it. When I look at the future and I think about the possibilities of getting back to that 10 again, I believe I can. Anything is possible. I really and truly believe that. In fact, my goal is an 11. Okay, realistically, maybe a 7 is the highest I will get in my life. Who knows for sure? But I do know this: if there is a chance I will make that 10 or 11, I will get there, because I will give it everything I have.

I know there are a lot of people in this world who have faced life-changing experiences like mine. And I can relate to the struggles they go through to live any kind of a normal life. There is no question that I know a great deal about that. To those people, I say this because I know it from experience: If you put your mind and your heart toward your goal, it is reachable with monumental effort. I believe that from the bottom of my heart.

I know that in difficult circumstances, it can appear to be a hopeless situation. Your prognosis is poor. There seems to be little chance for recovery. It's hard to summon even a single positive thought. I feel deeply for people who have encountered these kinds of situations because I have been there myself. There seems to be little reason to go on. I know all too well that feeling of hopelessness. You feel alone. You are unwilling to accept what has happened.

In those kinds of situations, I truly believe you have to embrace your faith. You might not be able to do anything physically, so the mental part is what you have to work on. And that is where faith can take over and provide you with the support you need.

Having God at your side is critical. It all begins in the head, with your thinking process. The physical part is important too, but it all starts with the mind. The mental part drives everything. You have to have your mind right before anything else can fall into place.

I said that to someone once, about the whole mental thing. And the response was a polite "How do you know that?" It wasn't a criticism, but an honest question. It was an easy answer for me to give. I would never have survived if I hadn't gotten my mind back on the right track. I never would have been able to apply myself to my physical recovery. I would have been stuck in despair. You have to begin to believe again. You have to know you will be able to do things again. Walk, talk, speak, eat. Yes, I will do all those thing again. That's in the mind. That is believing. And believing that God is at your side is the way it will work the best.

When I was in recovery, I encountered one problem after another. Infections. More surgeries. More backward steps. One serious problem after another. There was a period of time when my steps toward recovery were all going backward instead of forward. As my problems worsened, I was unable to think about my goals or keep in mind the positive things. It was all I could do to survive. There was not much room or time to think about the positives because, quite frankly, there weren't any. None! But I fought through it. I got my mind right incrementally. In the middle of the worst times, it was pretty hard to chart my strategy for recovery. But as I got better "What am I going to do about this?" became the central question. It is the question that propels me to take constant steps forward. I cannot tell you how important that statement is to me. For others who are struggling in any part of life, believe me: one step at a time. They add up.

Still, to this day, the thought never leaves me. Take my balance, for example. I know I have to get better at that. So what am I going to do about it? Exercise. Practice. Repeat. I used to draw a line on the ground and walk it over and over, keeping my balance. It wasn't much different from the field sobriety test you see police give to drunk drivers. *Sure, I can walk a straight line, Officer.* Mind you, I never had to take the police test. To regain my balance, I started slow. I was basically working at putting one foot in front of the other and moving forward. I did it over and over and over. Once I got a little more steady, I started running. I worked on a treadmill and on occasion utilized a water treadmill, which is very effective at improving muscle tone. I also did some rehab on a machine that stimulates the muscles through DC electrical current.

Sticking to a program and a stated goal is a good way to approach things. You can sink down to your lowest depths in life and feel sorry for yourself, or you can pull yourself up, ask yourself "What are you going to do about this problem?" and then do it.

Now, it may not always work. It didn't for me. When I started to learn to walk again, I could not even stand up on my own. So what was I going to do about it? Well, obviously, I didn't just bolt out of bed and run down the hall. But having my mind right on track with those thoughts was a good start, and it kept me going every day.

There have been so many situations I tackled this way. I really do ask this of myself repeatedly. And then I focus my attention on the specifics of what it is I will do to get to my goal. I don't expect it to just happen because I want it to. Life does not work that way. I know I will have to work on it. My goal to get back to normal is not just to improve but to get 100 percent perfect. I may never get there, but I will never give up; that is the crux of my thinking. *Positive. Positive. Positive. Practice. Practice. Practice.* It cannot be any other way.

Mental and spiritual strength is the foundation for getting through the toughest times. I look at myself and know I have made peace with God. He is at my side and I am comforted by this. We have come to terms with my situation and it gets me through each day. It is a lot better than being angry every day. After all, what purpose does that serve?

It is not easy to get through some things. As I said, you can't just get up and walk again. It may take an extraordinary amount of time to get to where you want to be, with enormous setbacks along the way. But you must always try to move ahead. I have, and it is a great feeling. The bottom line to all of this is that no matter what the hurdle, no matter what the obstacle, you must have your mind in the right place. You must never give up. I guess those are some pretty good thoughts to keep in mind. They sure work for me.

Duke Is Our Hero

The Pieper Family

Liz Pieper, Duke's Mother

Growing up, Duke was highly energetic and extremely determined. He started to walk when he was a little over eight months old. He didn't have skates on with those first steps, but I suppose if we had had skates on him, he would have skated, too. He was just that way.

Mark was in the heavy equipment business, and Duke wanted to be like his dad. We would throw dirty clothes down the steps from upstairs and then Duke would take his loader and load up the clothes in his dump truck and then drive the clothes over to the washing machine. We played those kinds of games constantly. He loved it and thrived on it from an early age.

He was involved in many sports as a kid. He played soccer, baseball, track-and-field, football, and then eventually got into hockey. Duke was a very good athlete and was quite tall for his age. With the hockey, though, he really didn't play at first. He learned to skate as a figure skater. I have a background in figure skating and have been an instructor for many years, running skating schools. Duke did actual figure skating in the beginning. He did ice shows and became an exceptional skater before he even learned any of the skills that go along with hockey. A couple times, Duke and our daughter, Jackie, even did ice show duets together.

Through all this, he really learned the basics of skating before he put the stick in his hand to eventually begin puck handling. Typically kids will focus their attention more on the puck handling and shooting part of the game rather than on the foundation of learning how to be a good skater first. Duke went in the opposite direction and learned the valuable skating skills before anything else.

Around the fourth grade, we noticed that from time to time he had headaches. He also had some trouble with such things as spelling. Then, at age 12, when Duke was playing Peewee hockey, he had this one game when he kept falling all the time. Duke was an exceptional skater and he never fell, so we couldn't figure out what was going on. His coach came up to us and said his skates must be dull and we should get them sharpened. But even after getting the skates sharpened, he still kept falling and falling. I recall Duke came up to me and told me he thought he might have an ear infection and this was what was causing the balance problems. I was not convinced because he had no other symptoms.

At that point, we really had no idea what was causing the problem, so Mark took Duke to the emergency room to have him examined. The diagnosis was some kind of inner ear problem, which did not sit right with me at all. Within a couple days, his vision became an issue. He started to see doubles of everything. At this point we all started thinking maybe he had a concussion. We had a different pediatrician take a look and she thought a concussion was a possibility—however, we could not recall a time when he hit his head that could have caused it.

Based on the concussion theory, the doctor said to play it that way, to have him take it easy. But this didn't sit well with me either. I thought we should get this checked out further. I took him to my ear, nose, and throat specialist for a full checkup. I told the doctor he was having double vision and that Duke felt as if something was in his ear. I wanted a thorough examination. They did a CT scan and told us Duke was bleeding in his brain. Right from there, we went to the emergency room at Abbott Northwestern Hospital. He was admitted and given an MRI.

Apparently there was so much blood that the MRI could not really tell what was happening at the time. We were sent home and referred to another doctor, who finally determined through a further exam that Duke had a cavernous hemangioma of the brain stem. It was down low on the brain stem, and we were told there was nothing that could be done at the time. Apparently the nerve damage caused by the bleed was what had caused the double vision. The thinking was that with time this would go away.

It took quite some time for the vision to get back to normal, about four months total. Duke was not able to do much of anything because he had the double vision the entire time. While waiting for his vision to clear, Duke basically did nothing except for some schoolwork. It was very difficult for him and for all of us. Around the four-month mark, the double vision cleared up and he was able to resume normal activities again. Then, that spring, he was able to get back into the flow. Things went well for a couple years, with no reoccurrence.

In the ninth grade, Duke transferred to Hill-Murray and made the varsity hockey team, which was quite an accomplishment for a freshman player. The night of the first game was going to be quite a special night for all of us. Duke was going to be playing his first varsity high school hockey game. Mark was at the arena in Burnsville and I was home with several friends and family, set to watch the game on television. It was that big of a game that it was being televised.

I noticed right away as the game started that Duke was not on the ice. I can recall thinking, *Why isn't he on the ice? What's wrong?* I'm trying to recall the exact sequence of events that took place, but I think I called my husband, Mark, and asked why Duke wasn't playing in the game. He told me Duke couldn't see and that his double vision had returned. He told me Duke had taken himself off the ice.

Mark took him right to the emergency room. I just knew as soon as I heard this that Duke's brain had started bleeding again. After some initial misdiagnoses and several consults with doctors, Duke was hospitalized a few days later.

Initially, we did not know the graveness of his situation. We had gone for some tests on a Friday and had actually planned to go out for breakfast after the evaluations. We were going to get the test results and then do what we had to do treatment-wise. Once we got the results and understood what was happening, it was overwhelmingly devastating.

I could not believe all this was happening to our son. I was absolutely scared to death. All I could think about on that Friday was, *I could lose my son. I could actually lose my son.*

After the surgery, I was elated. I thought it was over. I was so premature in my thinking. I just thought, *They took it out. It's fixed. We can move on. He is going to be okay. We don't have to worry about this anymore. No more bleeding.* I was so relieved, so incredibly overjoyed. I had no idea what was coming, what was ahead for each of us.

It was soon after that, that all the complications began. He got meningitis, and the effects were monumental. He had a horrible time, months of not knowing what was going on. He was completely out of it. He had severe nightmares. He thought he was playing hockey right there in his hospital bed. He would be kicking and turning and not knowing where he was. He would be up all night swatting bugs, sweating, and on and on. It was awful. The worst feeling in the world was the feeling of not being able to help my son. I could not help him and I was supposed to be there for him and help him. There was nothing I could do for him. Nothing.

We were basically living at the hospital. I cannot remember a time when one of us was not there with Duke, and I do not remember us leaving the hospital during that first month at all. Maybe I did, but I honestly don't think so.

Just when we would think he was getting better and on some kind of road to recovery, he would have one setback and then another. Infections in different places, rehab because he was improving, and then more problems, setbacks again, over and over. I honestly don't know how he made it through. He just never gave up. He never stopped fighting. Never.

When the infection went to his spine, it paralyzed him. There was a point when we thought Duke was not going to survive. As hard as it is to say, there was an actual time when we did not know if he was going to make it.

It was hard to even talk about what he went through during those incredibly difficult days. It was more than you would think any one person could bear in their life. I recall there were times when he was in the hospital following setback after setback when we thought, *No more.* We could not possibly take any more bad news and then it would come again and again and again. I learned one thing as a result of this and that is when you think you cannot take one more bad thing happening, the fact is you can take it, and move on.

We eventually brought Duke home to be homeschooled. We had an occupational therapist, a physical therapist, teachers, nurses, all there to help Duke. All these people were coming into the home to help him just get through the day. All of this had such a tremendous effect on Duke, and on the rest of us.

I can honestly say I don't remember almost a year of my daughter's life. I was gone all the time, every single day, with Duke. What was happening to him literally took over our entire lives. I'm not complaining here at all. It is just the way it had to be. Yet we were not there for our daughter. The Edina community took care of our daughter. She would stay with friends and some family, but for the most part during that year, we were not there for her. I feel terrible about it, but it had to be that way. I cannot say enough for the families that took her in and took care of her for us. I know it was all very hard on Jackie. What happened to Duke hit her very hard and for that period of time, almost a full year, all our lives changed dramatically.

Jackie got into hockey, and that's what got her through all the pain and agony that was present in our family. She never talked about it much, but we all knew it was an extremely hard time for her.

It was amazing how the school systems in Edina and at Hill-Murray pulled together to get Duke through the homeschool years so he could eventually return to Hill-Murray. I cannot say enough for the work the teachers did with and for him. They were absolutely wonderful. It was very important to Duke that he be able to graduate on time with his class. He worked so hard to make this happen, even though Mark and I were not totally ready for all that he was accomplishing. It was almost too much after all that had happened to him. He went to school, took online courses, and was absolutely determined to make graduation happen.

To graduate and at the same time face what he was going through cannot be put into words. He was on antibiotics, he had paralysis in his face on the left side, he had trouble eating and swallowing, and yet he moved ahead with school. It was just simply unbelievable.

Still, Duke was frustrated. He was embarrassed by his physical appearance. He had trouble with his eye and it required treatment. It stayed open all the time. But no matter what, he just kept going and going and going.

The prognosis for his face and eye was not good. We had to do something in order to keep him from losing his eye. Because the eye would stay open all the time, we had to continually use a gel to keep it from getting scratches. He needed surgery to save the eye and we were also told that the paralysis in his face would get worse and the side of his face would fall and close his breathing on that side. He had the plastic surgery where they took muscles and tendons out of his leg in order to pull everything up. And then the next surgery was to grow nerves across, from the other side of his face. The whole process was so involved, and yet Duke wanted it. He continued to battle and strive for normalcy.

Duke was and still is absolutely amazing. It is unthinkable what he has gone through, what he has overcome and how he has persevered. He never gave up and he still fights every day. He will make something of himself and of his life, and he will tell you that. He has a determination beyond anything you can imagine.

I could never begin to express everything Duke has gone through. I am so proud of him for how he has handled the whole situation and for how he has overcome all his obstacles. He is my role model. I wish I could be more like him. He has taken on every challenge that has confronted him. Most people will never in their entire lives face what Duke has faced already at this young age. He keeps going. I don't know what keeps him going. I don't know where his strength comes from, but it is there. I aspire to be like that person who he is and I am not and never will be.

Duke believes what happened to him was supposed to happen for a reason. I know that it has changed the dynamics of our entire family. It changed the way we look at things in life, how we perceive things and how we handle them.

He has made us appreciate the small things in life. He has made us sort out what is really important to think about and worry about. He has taught us about life, about never giving up. There may be times when life hits you in the face and you want to give up because you cannot handle any more. Well, you can. Duke has proven that to us and he continues to prove it every day.

We faced tortuous times when he was in the hospital and we wanted to give up and let Duke go. There were times when we felt it was time to let him go, give up. We thought we were fighting a losing battle. And yet, he kept battling to live and survive.

We owe so much to our family, friends, community, schools, teachers, hospitals, doctors, nurses, therapists, and all those who were there and pulled for us and for Duke. There will never be words to express how we feel about all of them. We could not have made it without their love and support.

We almost lost our wonderful son, but he is with us and inspires us each and every day of his magnificent life.

• • •

Jackie Pieper, Duke's Sister

When we were young, Duke and I were extremely competitive, as we are today. We always tried to win against each other in everything we did. It didn't matter what it was; we each wanted to win. With that kind of competitive spirit, the games and contests we had were very challenging.

Unfortunately, as we got older, it seemed as if we never really had the opportunity to spend much time together. First, Duke was gone playing hockey at Shattuck–St. Mary's. Then he had his serious injury, which went on for a long time. Now he is gone again, at Bowling Green. And when he is home for the summer or on breaks, it seems like I am gone, involved in something.

Duke was always interested in hockey. He was a really good player and very popular. He always had a lot of girlfriends and was a real leader among his friends. He has always had a great personality and liked to kid around a lot. This was true before his medical problems and still is today. He likes to make people feel good through his joking around. He is really good at it, too.

He has gotten into physical fitness even more than he was before, which is amazing to me after all he has been through. Church and religion has become a bigger part of his life as well. I think what happened to him has turned him in that direction in a positive way. It is also incredible to me that he has maintained his good spirits despite it all. His attitude is always good and he seems to find a way to look at the positives in life rather than the negatives.

Duke cares about people and is very respectful of others. He has a "never give up" attitude that was certainly a contributing factor in his recovery. My brother is a strong person. When I think about all he has gone through I cannot believe what he has accomplished and how much he has succeeded in his life.

If I were to say something to him that kind of summarizes my overall feelings about the past couple decades of our lives together, I would say to him, "Duke, I am so very proud of you. And I want you to know that I am very honored to call you my brother."

• • •

Mark Pieper, Duke's Father

When Duke was a youngster, I would bring him to work with me all the time. He especially liked to be around heavy equipment. He was fascinated by it. Bulldozers, those kinds of things were very much in his line of interest. Once he started school, it was sports. This gave me another opportunity to spend time with Duke. We were constantly trying to find ways to compete with one another. It was always who could kick the ball the farthest, who could pass the best, who could catch the best, hit the ball the farthest...always those kinds of competitive things. He loved it and I loved it. We were at each other all the time, too. He would make fun of me if I missed the ball and I would make fun of him. He was such a good kid and I had a great time around him.

Duke was pretty laid back when he was young. I can remember him playing soccer and standing around with his hands behind his back. We were together a lot, and it was really important to me that he had a good time. I guess it was why I would playfully tease him all the time. I wanted him to enjoy what we were doing. Even when he was young enough to be in a high chair, I can recall deliberately hitting the back of his elbow so he would spill the peas he had on his spoon, those kinds of things. And we would laugh and laugh. I still kid with him every chance I get.

I know that dads always think their kid is the greatest, but Duke really was a good player. He was an excellent skater because of my wife working with him at an early age. With her background in figure skating, she was able to start him at a very young age to learn the basics of skating, which put him ahead of most of the other kids.

I can recall being so proud of him when he made the Hill-Murray varsity hockey team, an accomplishment quite rare for a freshman. And then the first game came and it all started.

Once I found out how sick he was and what he was facing, it was devastating. In the beginning I thought only about what I hoped was the positive. I thought maybe he would miss a few games, a few weeks of school, and then get back to the routine. Even at different times when things started to go badly, I always kept in my mind that *Now, this isn't going to last long. Just give it a few more weeks and he will be back in school and we will get back to normal again.* And then we would have a setback. And then another setback. And another and another and another. From that point on he got worse and worse and worse and worse.

When you are going through something like this you are only able to see what is happening at the moment. Today we can look back and see the whole picture. There was one period when he was completely paralyzed from his toes to his neck. I am a religious person, and remember praying that maybe God could find a way to help Duke by giving him movement in his legs so he could someday walk and not live his life in a wheelchair. Then another time I thought, maybe if he could just get arm movement, he could feed himself. I was hoping for anything to get him out of his state of paralysis. I just wanted him to get a piece back here and a piece back there.

I can recall the day when the doctor gave us very little hope. The machine that was keeping him breathing was going to be shut off. I talked to Duke about what was happening. We had had enough at that point and could not see putting Duke through any more pain and discomfort. It was time.

I don't know how we coped with that thought. Who are we to judge when it is time to let someone you love die? Am I supposed to go to Duke and say, "Okay, this is enough now. It's time to die"? Or am I supposed to leave all of it up to God? I don't know. I didn't know. Another thought I had was maybe because of all the setbacks and the worsening condition, maybe this was a message from God that it was time. *How do we sort all this out? Are we keeping him alive for our own selfishness?* No one was there to tell us what to do.

All those thoughts ran through my mind, and yet the pain and suffering our son was going through was too much to bear, so we made the decision. But Duke wasn't ready. He did not want to die on a Wednesday. He wanted to stay alive and if he was going to die, for some reason, he wanted it to be on a Friday, not a Wednesday. I remember him telling me, "Dad, keep me alive until Friday and then let me die."

So we kept him going. Then Thursday night, by some kind of miracle, he got better. It had been one of our lowest moments to see him worsening by the day. He was drowning with no life jacket in sight, and then suddenly he improved some. He fought and fought. He never gave up.

Thinking back to those days, I would never have imagined in a million years that he would have gotten back to the point where he is today. I mean, there was a time when he could not hold his head up and could not do a single thing on his own—and yet he made it. He made it back to school, graduated with his class, and prepared for a college career.

I have my son and he is alive. I text him every day and still kid around with him as much as I can. I am so proud of him. I believe we are as close as ever, maybe closer. I look at him and what he went through and there is no doubt in my mind that he is my hero. I could never have gone through what he went through. When I was in college I broke my leg playing football, and I still have a limp because as it turned out one leg is shorter than the other. I was too embarrassed to wear a lift. I think about that. I was too embarrassed to wear a lift! And I look at my son and what he has faced every single day and how he has met his disabilities head-on.

Duke is unique. He never gave up. He survived. With all that he went through, I only saw him have somewhat of a breakdown on two occasions. We were told to be prepared for it to happen often, yet it didn't. On those brief occasions, it was more of a frustration that surfaced when Duke had to ask me to help him and do something for him because nothing was working up to that point. It was brief and to the point and lasted a short time only. And that was it. The rest he did himself. With me, when I got to the point of not being able to go on, I would go to the restroom and cry my eyes out and then come out with a smile on my face.

After going through all this, I know there is a God in this world. There is a higher power. I want people by reading this book to know that. I want them to know that there are miracles in this world because Duke is living proof that they exist. He has no business being here. He should not have survived. I know that my son is not afraid of death even though he came so close to it.

Once, during one of the worst times, I recall him saying to me, "Dad, they say heaven is so great, so what is so bad about getting there early to see what it is all about?" I told him, "Duke, I don't want you to go yet because I will miss you too much." He said, "Dad, you won't miss me because I will be right with you, right on your shoulder every single day." Think about that. I do. All the time.

CHAPTER 12

Life's Lessons

When I look back on my life so far, where do I begin? I was supposed to die. I was not supposed to be here. But I *am* here, and I have so much to say about what I have learned over the past few years. I want to pass it on. I want to share the lessons in life that I have come to understand. I have changed, no question about that.

My hopes, my dreams, and all that consumed me at the age of 15 changed in an instant, forever. I missed out on many great opportunities. I never had the chance to see how good of a hockey player I could become. I never had the chance to experience what most kids my age do. Athletics, routine educational opportunities, hanging out with my friends—regular teenager stuff eluded me.

I made the varsity at Hill-Murray School as a freshman, but I never played a single regular-season game. My dream of becoming an elite high school hockey player pursued by colleges never came to fruition. My goal of being a collegiate hockey star was never realized. My pursuit of a career in the National Hockey League, and someday skating around the ice holding the Stanley Cup, will never become a reality.

I have accepted this and moved on, after a lot of reflecting on my past and future. Imagine for a moment skating on the ice at an ice arena filled with cheering fans. Your skates are gliding along the ice as effortlessly as possible. Your blades cut sharply one way and then the other. Your stick connects dead-on with the puck and you watch it as it soars away from you, on its way to the goal. The round, black object gets smaller and smaller as it moves farther and farther away from you until you see it cut deeply into the back of the net over the sprawled opposing goalie. You score, and a magnificent rush pounds through your veins; the taste of satisfaction in your mouth is overwhelming. And to solidify the moment, you see the red light behind the net go on.

Now imagine yourself lying in a hospital bed, paralyzed from the neck down. You have a feeding tube stuck in your mouth. You are blind, catatonic, and you have no idea if you will even live through the day. Imagine having a 5 percent chance of survival. Imagine you cannot do even the simplest biological things and have to learn how to breathe again, eat again, swallow, walk, and talk. That was the beginning of my story.

I don't have much of a recollection of most of the early stuff. But then I guess it is probably for the best that I don't remember everything. I mean, what is the point? Why would I want to remember every detail of such a dark time? I feel fortunate that I retain so little from those days. But I do know this: I am here today because of a few miracles.

I do believe in miracles and am convinced I am living proof of their existence. By my definition, a miracle is something that occurs that is not supposed to occur. All odds are against it. The event or act is something so far out of the ordinary that it comes as a surprise to most who witness it. It is something that often brings joy and gratitude of the highest magnitude. If the story of my survival isn't a miracle, then I don't know what is.

I had my first brain bleed in 2006, but the doctors could not treat the condition or operate on me at the time. A second bleed occurred, just as predicted, approximately two years later. It was then that I came in close proximity to death. I continued, on the brink in a state of medical emergency, enduring several subsequent surgeries and procedures. I had various interventions over time, such as treating infections in my brain and spine, a shunt in my brain, a tracheotomy, feeding tubes, catheters, just to name a few. I suffered total temporary paralysis as I fought a battle to simply live. Surviving all that, I then faced the inability to do most of life's normal functions—breathing, swallowing, talking, walking, writing. I couldn't even brush my teeth. I had to begin again with the most elementary things.

By the time I left the hospital, I had regressed educationally to the fourth grade. Yet miracle of miracles: I graduated from high school—on time with my class. And I am on track to graduate with a college degree from Bowling Green State University, too.

Why me? It's a question I've asked myself in various ways over the past years. Is it all a bad thing? No, absolutely not. Sure, if given the choice I would never have wanted it to happen to me—or anyone else, for that matter. It changed my life forever. I will never play hockey again and will likely never be completely normal to do the things in life I used to be able to do without any thought or effort.

Yet what happened did change me for the better. I *know* I am a better person. I am more concerned about others, more thankful for what I have, and more motivated to live a well-rounded life. I am more patient with other people and my friendships are much more abundant. I have broadened my horizons. Life is good. I'm happy. Today I look at life in a very different way. I feel good about myself and I am endlessly proud of what I have accomplished. That might seem difficult to believe, but it's true. I really do feel that way.

Early on it was very difficult for me. Looking back on some of my journal notations from that time put it into perspective for me:

> *November 15, 2012 (Almost four years after my initial surgery in December 2008): I have accepted that I'm messed up. I got face injuries and I just don't look like everyone else but I accept it. I love the guy who I am for me, even though I might be different in one way or another.*

• • •

> *December 28, 2012: It's just so hard looking at the television and finding world junior hockey players on the air. That's where I should be instead of sitting on my butt watching.*

• • •

> *December 30, 2012: I was watching that man preach, and what really stood out to me is it's an insult to God when we wish that we were like someone else. Everyone was created to be their own masterpiece.*

• • •

January 13, 2013: You haven't lost your dream. Jesus says the thing against you is that you have not gone after that dream. That's when I was made to pick up the broken pieces from the floor and turn them into something great.

• • •

January 29, 2013: Keep moving on and forget about the past and move forward. Work on getting that body in shape. Focus on the small goals and you will make something out of your life still.

• • •

January 30, 2013: I want to be proud of what I've done. I am not proud when I tell people I had a life-changing experience. I gotta fix that...I will fix that!

• • •

January 31, 2013: Where do you want your life to go? I still want to play in the National Hockey League. That's still in my head that I can make it. But sometimes I have to face the fact that that's not reality. I know I have to face the fact.

• • •

February 7, 2013: It's another one of those nights. I feel it coming on even before I feel the full effects. I just know it is a helpless feeling and I know there is absolutely nothing I can do to stop this from happening. I feel like I am beating myself up inside and

I just want to take myself outside and punch away at myself for letting my dreams get away from me. It is so hard living with myself, knowing that my body has left me. I'm not the type of person, when opportunities come my way, to let them get away. I have always taken advantage of them and I feel like I let myself down. I never do that because it is against what my heart and soul stand for in life. It takes every ounce of my energy to prevent myself from putting my fist through a window. I am so disappointed in myself, in my body, and I know I will never be able to explain to anyone how I feel. In the past, when adversity came my way I would always find a way to fight through it. That's what I have always done and it is so hard to accept that a pea-sized ball of blood did this to me. It is so sad to me just remembering some of the things that my body used to be able to do before all this happened. Too many thoughts, too many hopes...gone.

I have said many times that I don't dwell on the past. *Keep moving ahead. If you don't like how you feel, then do something about it.* My journal entries do confirm, however, that simply saying "it is all forgotten" is nothing more than a pipe dream. I will likely always experience setbacks and disappointments, but hopefully only momentary, as these were. They do not detract from my mission to move ahead, accept what has happened, and learn from it. I can. I do and I will.

If someone were to assess why certain people have satisfying careers and are basically happy, good-natured people, I truly believe it all starts with one thing: attitude. Attitude is the center of just about everything we do, especially if we are measuring how we feel on a given day or how we look at the future. If you are going to evaluate how your life is going, take a close, hard look at your overall attitude. I have, and there is a time in my life, looking back, that I am not proud of; I'm not proud of who I was.

The debilitating brain bleed that created a major change in my life most importantly changed my attitude. My attitude toward people, my circumstances, and life in general has changed dramatically. It really has.

I feel that I was truly saved by the grace of God—saved from dying more than once, saved from paralysis, saved from a life in a wheelchair...so many other things. I will not waste those miracles that were granted to me. I intend to assist others who face similar or major life changes. I likely will always have some rough days and nights when I think about what could have been. But when those moments sneak up on me, what gets me through it is my faith and my positive attitude. They prop me up in even the most difficult times.

Before I truly was of the belief that my future rested in playing hockey. I know that won't happen, but hockey can still be a part of my life. I just don't know how, where, or in what capacity. It is no longer the center of my universe, but I think there is still room for it.

I faithfully believe that what God has started in my life, He will finish. He will not leave me alone to find my own way. He will not forget about me and leave me to struggle in the dark. And this thought is what gets me through every day of the week, month, and year. I need this assistance. I need to believe that everything is going to be all right in my life. It's interesting and yet frustrating at the same time because so much of my recovery has been rehabilitation and therapy, and those kinds of things focus on the physical part of it. The other side, the mental part of it, had little effect until I decided to do it on my own with God's help.

The lingering thought is, *What happens next? What will I have to face in the future? More problems? More infections? Another bleed?* Although I have improved dramatically from where I began, how much I will improve remains a big question for me. Will I ever lose my double vision? Will I continue to be able to drive a car? Will I be able to skate again? Handle a puck on the ice? I truly believe I will, and as I have said many times over, I will never give in until I have achieved my goals.

So what's next? Well, I think it is quite easy to figure out, probably easier to figure out than actually accomplish, but here goes: You accept what you have, alter your dreams, and make the new plan work. It sounds quite simple. And I truly believe it is. I will find my niche. Maybe it will be in hockey—scouting, coaching, or perhaps as an analyst or a commentator. Who knows? But I do know that I love the game, and with my passion and desire I will find my way.

Someone once asked me a really tough question about hockey and I can honestly say I am not sure of my answer, then or now. The question was, "If hockey was and continues to be so special to you, and you often refer to what happened to you as an injury, then why are you not angry with the game? Why is it still such a big part of your life?"

It is a great question. I still don't know how to answer it. I have never been mad at the game. It's a part of me. I love it. When all this happened to me, I was mad at God, mad at my parents, mad at life, mad at myself, and generally a despondent, angry kid in every possible respect. But I was *never* mad at hockey, even though playing the game is what likely caused my injury to begin with. (I have always felt that my brain bleed occurred because of an earlier head injury I received playing hockey. My dad thinks that might be the case, too, and even recalls a specific game when he suspects it might have occurred. For the record, my mom feels differently; she thinks I may have been born with this issue that later caused the problems. I seriously don't know and I don't think anyone ever will. In the end, it doesn't matter. It happened, and there isn't a thing I can do about it. It is what it is. I am what I am. So let's move on.)

Maybe that's my answer: I just don't have an answer. All I know is I will always love the game of hockey. I know I will want to continue with the game because it has brought so many wonderful things to my life. This takes nothing away from my family and friends and all the joy they have brought to my life, but the game occupies a huge part of my heart and soul, even today.

The game has given me so many positive things. Since that fateful day I left the ice, not for one hour, one minute, or one second have I had that wonderful experience of playing hockey again. And perhaps I never will, but the pure pleasure and love for the game will never escape me. Hockey has been and remains the love of my life. I think it always will be. If I'm not involved in it professionally, I know I will watch the game as a fan and continue to enjoy every aspect of it. I have very little doubt about that.

I think for the most part I am in pretty good physical and mental shape given what I have gone through. I focus my motivation on attending classes and keeping up a good grade-point average. My goal is to graduate on time, in four years. I want to keep the good relationships with my professors at Bowling Green. I also maintain my close connection with my family even though they are many miles away. I enjoy hanging out with my friends, and still feel that team camaraderie with the hockey team. Even though I am not playing, I watch a lot of games on TV.

Educational success is at the top of my agenda, but having fun is a priority, too. Second to school on my agenda are my workouts. Keeping my body in the best possible condition is as important to me now as ever. I want to be able to present myself well to others in the classroom. I want to function as normally as possible, even with the multiple accommodations that are in place for me. I continue to do everything in my power not to let my disabilities stand in my way and stop me from doing what I want to do.

Sometimes I struggle, but that's okay, because I will always work my way through it. I remember one class that was a particular challenge for me. It involved a lot of note-taking, and that tripped me up mightily. It took a lot of extra work to keep up, but I managed to pass the class. It sure helped that my teacher was very responsive to my needs. When there were things I could not keep up with, I got the help I needed after classes, during office hours. That helped me immensely. In some of my classes I would have someone do the note-taking for me, one of the educational accommodations BGSU allowed me. No matter the roadblock, I will do everything in my power to find a way around it.

I'll admit that as positive as I am, life is no bed of roses—not by any stretch of the imagination. My toughest times come at night, about once a month, when I am overcome with feelings of deep depression. I can tell when it is coming, and yet I cannot pinpoint the actual reasons that bring this state of mind on. It never lasts very long, usually just through the night until I fall asleep, and when I wake up then I feel better. But in the midst of that feeling, I feel deep sorrow and self-pity. My mind races and races. I'm seized with "what-ifs" and recriminations. Thankfully, I am getting better at coping with these moments. Time heals all wounds.

My workouts keep my frame of mind where I want it to be, most of the time. I call that positive mind-set my "happy place." When I go to my happy place, my mind literally goes blank of anything other than pure enjoyment. I get there a lot now.

Hockey did that for me when I played it. Those were my happiest moments. I used to get so lost in the game that I was in a sort of dreamland for hours. The adrenaline rush was superior to anything else I had ever experienced. It is going to take time, but I truly believe I will find that sort of bliss once again.

As I look for my calling, the most important thing is to realize the tremendous power of the human mind. It can do so much for a person, both physically and mentally. Its power is absolutely unbelievable. The mind tells the body what to do. It can reinforce the positive and have so much control over the negative as well. I am living proof of that. No matter what a person's situation, one's state of mind is critical. I know from my own experience that getting my mind on the right track was a crucial step in regaining my normalcy. I would not have gotten through otherwise.

In addition, I have to give my parents so much of the credit. I learned from my mom about being the glue that holds everything together. She knows what has to be done and she gets it done. She is a rock when it comes to covering every last detail. And my dad provides me with the motivation I need. *Move ahead, never give up, never quit—work, work, work.* His work ethic is second to none. My parents complement each other and provide great balance for our family. They each motivate and inspire me in their own ways. I want them to be pleased and proud when they see the improvements I make and the path I am taking toward a normal, productive future. So far, I believe I have done them proud.

There was a time in my life when I felt like giving up. There didn't seem to be a point. I was a mess with little hope on the horizon. It was a bad time. After all, I was supposed to die. And at the time, I honestly didn't care. It all seemed so hopeless. I was destined to a life of misery and I could not stand it anymore.

But I lived! I altered my fate. I fought. I rebelled against the destruction that had been done to my body. With God's assistance, I have been given a second chance at life—and believe me, I do not want to screw it up.

I have gone from the depths of despair to feeling really optimistic about the future. There was a reason for all this. I haven't quite figured it all out yet, but I will. I hope I can provide some guidance and inspiration to others who face their own hardships. Know this: You are not alone. Others have suffered like you are suffering. But you can make it through. As hard as it may seem, you can make it through. I believe in you, like so many others believed in me.

There will be times when the darkest days get even darker. Just when it seems like nothing in the world can be so bad, it will get worse. And it is in those times that you must march ahead. Rise above it all and stay in the fight. NEVER give in. You have to believe. You have to always take the high road, think positively, and look for the light at the end of the tunnel. It is there. You just have to find it. I did and I am still following it.

I have learned and am living proof that there is a path to normalcy, and I am on it. It is beautiful—with hopes, dreams, and love abounding at each step as I move ahead. My journey begins anew every day, and the lessons I have learned have become imbedded in my heart and deep in my soul.

Thank you for taking the time to join me.

Strategies for Survival

There is no question that I have had a difficult journey, but I have already come so far. There is no time to dwell on the past, only time to make every effort to move forward toward the future. I had a lot of help getting here, and have looked for inspiration wherever I could find it. There are three quotes in particular that have resonated with me, and I've committed them all to memory.

> *"It's not whether you get knocked down, it's whether you get back up."*
>
> —*Vince Lombardi*

> *"The ultimate measure of a man is not where he stands in moments of comfort and convenience, but where he stands at times of challenge and controversy."*
>
> —*Martin Luther King Jr.*

> *"The true measure of your worth includes all the benefits others have gained from your success."*
>
> —*Cullen Hightower*

In addition, I created a sort of blueprint for how I want to live my life. These strategies have aided immeasurably in my progress. I hope they will inspire others who face difficult journeys, too.

- Nothing is out of reach. Philanthropist T.F. Buxton once said, "With ordinary talent and extraordinary perseverance, all things are attainable." I was blessed with extraordinary talent as an athlete and young hockey player. Then, without even a moment's notice, it was taken from me. I was left paralyzed, given a 5 percent chance of living, and rendered unable to do life's simplest things. But I have persevered— and I have learned that even the most seemingly unattainable things are within reach.

- Feeling bad today? What are you going to do about it? Believe me, I still have some pretty bad days every once in a while. And when I have one of those days, I ask myself the question, *Do I like how I feel today?* When the answer is no, the response to myself is simple: *Well, what are you going to do about it?* With that question, I am able to move on.

- Forget the negative and think positively! What possible good does it do to think about the negatives in your life? None. I like to think about the positives. If you do, you will never go anywhere complaining about your life or feeling sorry for yourself. You have to be content with whom God made you to be today. I think about where I started in my recovery and where I am today. I think about being happy and enjoying what I have. Focusing on the positive keeps your mind right. It's that mind-over-matter thing. It works!

- Be thankful to God for what you have. A few short years ago, I was paralyzed and completely helpless; I couldn't even breathe on my own. Now I'm going to college at Bowling Green State University. I can drive, help out with the hockey program, and I maintain a B average. I have a lot of friends, a loving family, and am looking forward to the future. I am very thankful. I was at war with God for a brief time. I didn't understand; I couldn't accept what had happened to me. Now I do. God has been with me—holding me up, counseling me. We are best friends again, and I am grateful.

- Keeping your body in shape gets the rest of you in shape. Staying physically fit has always been a priority for me, and in recovery it has been a tremendous motivational tool. It is something I can look forward to every single day. When I am in great physical condition, it bolsters my attitude toward everything. It provides an overwhelming positive in my life.

- Mind over matter. For me, this strategy is an important part of my existence. I have to have my mind right. It gets me to where I want to go and brings me out of even my darkest moments. It is nothing less than the foundation for peace in life.

- Look around. It's not as bad as you think. Feeling bad about yourself today? Well, take a look around and I guarantee you, you will find someone worse off than you are. So instead, count your blessings. I take stock, and do a count every day. There are so many things to be thankful for if you look for them. So try to do that instead of looking for the things that you're not happy about.

- Set mental and physical goals. I know where I was after my first surgery and the many that have followed. I'm doing more now and have surpassed the expectations of family, friends, doctors, and everyone else. And I'm not finished yet. I have a lot left to do, and I do not plan to waste time getting to where I want to be.

- Be an inspiration for others. This happened to me for a reason, and I am not going to let it go unnoticed. Every chance I get, I intend to be the type of person who can be an inspiration to those less fortunate than me (and even those more fortunate who don't know it yet). I will live my life and become a person worthy of admiration. Being able to share my story and be an example for positive change in someone else's life makes what happened to me worthwhile.

- Learn from each roadblock and setback. Roadblocks and setbacks are unavoidable; I have seen more than my fair share in the past few years. Yet I will not let them block my path to life's normalcy ever again. Each one is an opportunity to learn something, and overcoming them makes me stronger and stronger as I continue on my mission to recovery.

- Focus on the future. The future lies ahead of us. It is the next day, next week, next month, next year. For me, what comes with it is my education, my career, my family, and my friends. I only get one shot at it, so I will be giving it everything I have in order to make my life a success. When I look back someday, I want to be sure I have left nothing on the table, that I have given everything I have to be successful in my own eyes and in the eyes of those I care about.

- Ask yourself, "How am I doing?" Every so often, I have to do a self-evaluation—a report card, so to speak. *How am I doing?*

What do I need to improve on? Am I meeting my goals to this point? Am I on the right track? I want high marks and won't settle for anything less. Self-evaluation is an important aspect of moving forward. It's a way to chart overall progress, and something that keeps the adrenaline flowing. For me, it keeps my spirits up and paves the way for continual improvement in all areas I need to work on.

- Enjoy every day as the gift it is. Life is a precious gift, and it is important to recognize and appreciate it. I never let myself forget that. I do my best to find a way to enjoy every single day. I strongly believe that a person's attitude will be the key to success or failure in life. It will make you feel good or make you feel bad. It can control your thinking and your outlook during a second, minute, hour, day, month or year. It will keep you positive or negative. It is an easy decision to make: do you want to be miserable or happy? The way I see it, there is only one way to go.

- Be a positive force for others. I have said many times that there is a reason for all that has happened to me. I truly believe this. I have a mission to assist and help others who have also had life-changing experiences. Making a difference in others' lives is as important as anything that I do.

- Leave the past in the past. You cannot change the past, whatever it may be. No matter how much you would like to go back and have another chance to do it all over again, it will not happen. So look ahead. Look to the future and try to enjoy every moment of every single day. It will all be worth it.

ACKNOWLEDGMENTS

I am grateful to so many people who have helped me along my difficult journey. Frankly, I don't know where to begin—and certainly not where to end.

I have to start with my mom and my dad, who have fought my battle alongside me every single day since the first time we had any sense there might be a problem in my brain. I could fill pages upon pages with examples of what they have done for me, how they have supported me, guided me, advised me and mostly, through it all, just loved me.

If there was a fixed, absolute template for parenting, they have been the mold for it. Never wavering, never giving in, never being anything but the best parents they could be has been their practice for my entire life, especially the past six years. They have provided the guidance, support, and strength for me to get up in the morning and face each new day. They will never fully know how much I love them and how much I appreciate everything they have done for me. I cannot thank them enough.

My sister, Jackie, is the best. I am so grateful to her for weathering the storm along with me. I am so proud to call her my sister. Every guy should have a sister like Jackie, and they would then feel the wonderful sibling connection that I do. I love her for hanging in there with me.

To my countless relatives, doctors, nurses, hospital staff, teachers, coaches, former teammates, and friends: thank you. I have learned from you. I admire you. All of you have been my inspiration and fueled my spirit. My gratitude is everlasting.

—Duke

. . .

One thing I have always believed is that a person's attitude may be the most singular part of his personality that will determine his success or failure in his career, as well as in his personal life. Attitude seems to be at the forefront of just about everything we do. It controls how we feel, how we work, and most importantly whether or not we enjoy and give our very best in all facets of life.

When I think of Duke, what strikes me first is his attitude. Over the course of the last couple years, I have had the pleasure of being with him on numerous occasions as we worked on his book. Not for one second have I seen anything in him that falls short of being absolutely terrific in every respect.

Between the covers of this book is the story of a young man who had his whole life turned upside down. His passion for someday playing high school, collegiate, and perhaps even professional hockey was ripped from his grasp. His talent and unique abilities were torn from his body and soul. The sport he trained for and loved since he was a youngster fell away from him in a split second.

When Duke came off the ice during warm-ups to tell Hill-Murray hockey coach Bill Lechner that he could not play in his first varsity game, neither Duke, his coach, his family, nor anyone that knew him realized he would never go back on the ice—with his team or any team—again. Facing a slim survival rate, then paralysis, and having to learn all the basics in life over again was just the beginning.

His hopes and dreams had been crushed. It was more than most could ever bear, but for Duke it merely provided him with the motivation to understand and overcome his obstacles. He believes that it happened for a reason, perhaps to test his fortitude, his toughness, and to aid him in his new goal: to provide a platform to assist others facing life-changing experiences.

It has been an incredible honor to work with and get to know Duke. He is a wonderful human being with a huge heart, who has lived more of his life in the past 22 years than most of us will live in a lifetime.

Thank you to Duke and the Pieper family for allowing me to share in your story.

—Jim Bruton